Robert Winston is an internationally respected gynaecologist specializing in infertility. He is Director of the Infertility Clinic at Hammersmith Hospital, London, the largest comprehensive infertility clinic in the UK offering the test-tube baby treatment on the National Health Service.

He has been visiting Professor at the Universities of Texas and Leuven (Belgium) and Clyman Visiting Professor at the Mount Sinia Hospital, New York. His research has been in collaboration with leading infertility centres in the USA, Canada, West Germany and Belgium. He has written many specialist papers on infertility and holds the rare and prestigious post of Professor of Fertility in the University of London.

He presented the award-winning series *Your Life in Their Hands*, for BBC Television, and the BBC TV series *Making Babies* was devoted to the work of the Infertility Unit at Hammersmith.

Professor Winston is married with three children. He is now a member of the House of Lords and is active in advising on all matters on human reproduction.

INFERTILITY

A sympathetic approach to understanding the causes and options for treatment

Professor Robert M.L. Winston

MB, BS, FRCOG

Professor of Fertility Studies, University of London
Institute of Obstetrics and Gynaecology
Hammersmith Hospital, London

VERMILION
LONDON

To my wife Lira,
Who continually provides the love,
support and understanding which makes
this work possible.

First published in Great Britain Martin Dunitz in 1986
Revised editions published by Macdonald Optima in 1987 and by
Optima in 1994

1 3 5 7 9 10 8 6 4 2
Copyright © Robert M.L. Winston 1986, 1987, 1994, 1996

This edition published in the United Kingdom in 1996 by
Vermilion, an imprint of Ebury Press

Random House UK Ltd
Random House
20 Vauxhall Bridge Road
London SW1V 2SA

Random House Australia (Pty) Ltd
20 Alfred Street
Milsons Point Sydney
New South Wales 2016 Australia

Random House New Zealand Limited
18 Poland Road, Glanfield
Aukland 10 New Zealand

Random House South Africa (Pty) Limited
PO Box Bergvlei South Africa

Random House UK Limited Reg. No. 954009

A CIP catalouge record for this book is available from the British Library.

ISBN 0 09 181405 7

Printed and bound in Great Britain by Mackays of Chatham, plc

Papers used by Vermilion are natural, recyclable products from wood grown in
sustainable forests.

Contents

Acknowledgements

My greatest debt is to my patients whose bitter and sometimes sweet experience taught an imperfect pupil the basis for this book. I am grateful to many members of the Hammersmith team but in particular to Dr Masood Afnan, who read the manuscript at a critical stage and who made many helpful suggestions, to my secretary Mrs Josie Cronin whose intelligent and commonsense advice was very useful and to Jennifer Hunt, our infertility counsellor, who has helped crystallize many of the ideas in this book. I am also grateful to Mary Banks of Martin Dunitz, publishers, whose assiduous editorial work smoothed many rough corners off the first edition.

Lastly, I owe much to my close colleague Mr Raul Margara, without whose professional support and warm friendship this book would not have been written.

RMLW
1993

1

Identifying your problem

It surprises most people to learn that at least one in ten couples have a problem trying to conceive. Unfortunately, for many it is a very persistent condition and one that causes great feelings of longing or grief. If you have this difficulty, or if you or your partner think that you may have a problem in getting pregnant, then this book is primarily written for you. In recent years, there has been a large number of important advances in the treatment of infertility, and a bit more attention is now focused on the plight of people who are infertile.

The reason I have written this book is that, in the course of running a busy full-time medical practice devoted to problems of fertility, I find a huge number of men and women who feel that things have not been fully explained or discussed with them. So many people go through endless tests or what seem to be irrational treatments and get increasingly frustrated. Others despair because they cannot find out what the real chances of a pregnancy are. Many couples just want to know whether the newer treatments – such as the test-tube baby method – are for them. If you have had any of these worries, then I hope that this book may help.

It is written deliberately from a medical point of view. I have tried to be very truthful. No attempt has been made to hide when treatments are likely to be unsuccessful. Most people who are infertile need accurate information rather than false optimism.

When should I start worrying?

An average fertile couple having unprotected sex have about an 18 per cent chance of conceiving each month. Thus, about half the fertile population take about four to five months to conceive and most normal couples will have expected to have started a pregnancy within a year of trying to conceive. If after eighteen months of regular intercourse without contraception you haven't conceived you most probably have a problem. It is most important to realize that this is likely to be minor and that the majority of people need only fairly straightforward treatment to get pregnant.

There are certain pointers to the possibility of a fertility problem. These may encourage you to seek medical help before eighteen months have elapsed. If you think that you have one of the following problems and you want to get pregnant, it may well be worthwhile seeking your family doctor's advice after about six months of trying.

Your periods are infrequent   If you never have periods or if they come only at intervals of longer than two months, it may be that you are not ovulating regularly. This is usually easily treated (see page 44).

You have felt increasing pain with your periods or deep pain on intercourse   If you have recently noticed that your periods have become increasingly painful or that you get deep discomfort inside the vagina during intercourse, it may be that you have some infection in the pelvis (see page 54) or possibly endometriosis (page 74). It is worth asking for a prompt appointment with a gynaecologist if you have these symptoms.

You had a burst appendix or severe peritonitis in the past or had a definite infection at the time of an earlier pregnancy or miscarriage   It could just be that you have a problem with the tubes or even with the inside of the uterus. A gynaecologist may recommend early laparoscopy (a telescope inspection of your pelvis – see page 42) or an x-ray of the tubes. My feeling is that if you have had any suggestion of these kinds of problems in the past, you should at least talk to your doctor if you don't become pregnant within about six months.

You are over thirty-six years old   If you are a woman and getting towards your forties, you will be naturally less fertile. Actually, about one third of all normal women are subfertile by the age of forty. For example, they do not really need to use contraceptives if they don't want a pregnancy. The problem is that nobody can tell them whether they will be in the naturally infertile group of older women. The situation is similar if you are in your late thirties and trying to get pregnant. Because there is no way of knowing whether you are likely to become 'biologically' infertile fairly soon, it is worth getting tests done at an earlier stage, to maximize your chances of pregnancy as soon as possible.

WHAT CAUSES INFERTILITY?

Either the man or the woman may be infertile. Because infertility is so common, it often happens that an infertile man meets an infertile woman and both partners may contribute to the childlessness. Very roughly, the woman is the infertile one in about half of all infertile couples. In about 30 per cent of infertile couples, it is the man who has the main problem. In the remaining 20 per cent, both partners contribute equally.

To understand what causes infertility, we need to get a little technical. I make no apology for this, because it is only by appreciating what normally happens that we can really understand what has gone wrong. Let us look at how people get pregnant. What I think will surprise readers is how incomplete our knowledge sometimes is. From time to time I shall point out what we don't know. The fact that doctors and scientists do not know everything about how pregnancies are normally conceived may help explain why not all cases of infertility are understood either. If you find this part of the book boring, I suggest you come back later and read the bits of this part that seem relevant to your problems.

Essentially, getting pregnant involves the meeting of a sperm with an egg. The process is complex. To start with the sperm.

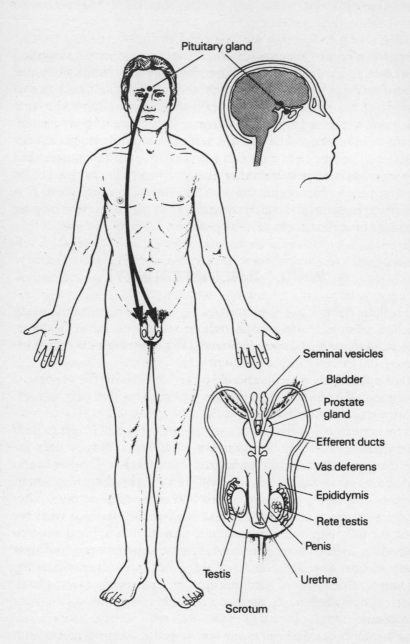

Pituitary gland

Seminal vesicles

Bladder

Prostate gland

Efferent ducts

Vas deferens

Epididymis

Rete testis

Penis

Testis

Urethra

Scrotum

The male reproductive organs

Sperm production

Spermatozoa, or sperms, are first produced at puberty. They are manufactured in the testis, the organ that hangs in the scrotum. The testis is filled with minute tubes inside which the sperm grow. Sperm manufacture requires a slightly lower temperature than the rest of the body and this may be why the testis hangs in the scrotum, which is about four degrees cooler than the temperature inside the abdomen. It is for this reason that men are sometimes advised to take regular cold baths if they are infertile, though this advice is of dubious value. After all, a man can't sit in a cold bath all day!

The minute tubes in which sperm grow in the testis are joined to more tubes, called the rete testis (see the diagram opposite). The rete testis is joined to yet more tubes, called the efferent ducts, of which there are usually about ten. Each one of these ducts is much finer than a thin piece of cotton. The efferent ducts all lead into a single tube, called the epididymis, which as you will see is a pretty extraordinary piece of plumbing. Sperm are not capable of fertilizing an egg if taken directly from the testis. To become functional they need to travel from the testis, through the tubing of the epididymis into the outside world.

The epididymis is a remarkably coiled tube about the thickness of a piece of button cotton. It is about twelve metres long and all the sperms travel through it. At the beginning of this journey the sperm are not motile – that is, they cannot swim. They are forced along this narrow passage probably by muscular contractions in the tube wall and possibly by hydrostatic pressure. The sperm are changed chemically in the epididymis so that by the end of their journey through it they are capable of swimming actively. The epididymis seems essential if these changes are to happen. The epididymis can become damaged by infection or injury and this can prevent normal development of sperm. Alternatively, it may become completely blocked, in which case no sperm can be produced. The journey just through the epididymis takes about fourteen days, depending partly on how often the man has sex.

The epididymis is joined to the vas deferens, another single tube. This is a thicker tube, about one-sixth of an inch (4 m) across and very muscular. It can just be felt in most men between finger and thumb in the region of the groin. During ejaculation, contractions in the vas (the plural is vasa, and there is one supplying each testicle) propel the sperm into the urethra. The urethra is the pipe that connects the bladder to the outside world via the penis. During this part of the journey taken by sperm, fluid is produced by the seminal vesicles, two reservoirs connected to the vasa, and by the prostate gland. This fluid goes to make up the total seminal fluid, in which sperm are bathed. It contains chemicals essential to sperm health. If the vesicles or prostate have been infected or damaged in some way, the man may be infertile.

Ejaculation occurs during the male orgasm. The muscles at the base of the penis pump the seminal fluid in spurts. The total volume of semen may vary from one millilitre to about eight millilitres (about one and a half teaspoonsful). If there is insufficient fluid, the man may be infertile; alternatively, too much fluid may dilute the sperm too much. On the whole, though, the precise volume is not all that important. Most of the sperm escape in the first spurt of the ejaculate. At ejaculation, the semen is jelly-like and the sperm are incapable of fertilization. The semen has to liquefy, a process that takes place automatically in normal men within about thirty minutes of ejaculation. Even then, the sperm may not be capable of fertilizing an egg. They need to undergo another chemical process, so-called capacitation, which takes place on contact with the woman's bodily fluids.

Egg production

When a little girl is born, her ovaries contain about two million eggs. These eggs have actually been present since a few weeks after conception. By the time she reaches puberty and starts to have periods, many of the eggs that she started life with will have disappeared. Curiously, out of all the eggs that were in her ovaries only about four to five hundred will ever be ovulated (shed from the ovary) and in most cases, out of the millions of eggs she started with only two or three will ever become children.

During childhood, a girl's ovaries are hardly active at all. The key to adult development is actually the pituitary gland in the brain. This is about the size of a large pea and lies under the centre of the base of the brain. It is the 'master' gland and to some extent

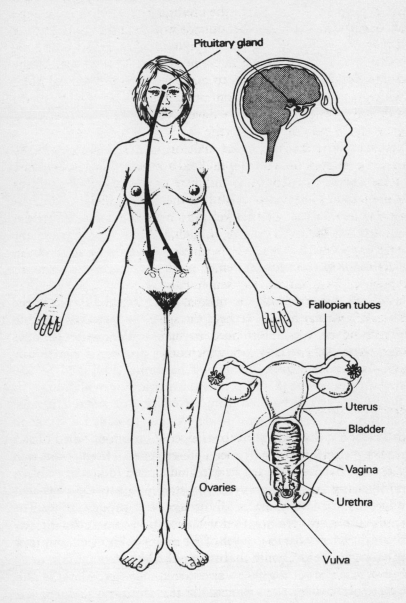

The female reproductive organs

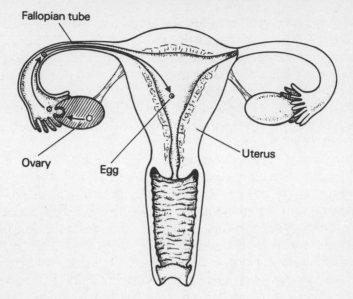

Egg formation and movement

controls all the other hormone glands (such as the thyroid in the neck). As the time for puberty approaches, the pituitary gland in the brain starts to send hormonal messages to the ovaries (in boys to the testicles). Precisely what starts this process is not understood. These hormones, luteinizing hormone (LH) and follicle stimulating hormone (FSH), pepare the ovaries for ovulation.

Before an egg can be shed from the ovary, or ovulated, it must be mature. The egg matures inside a structure called a Graafian follicle (see the diagram above), which is a little fluid-filled blister or cavity inside the ovary. The egg, which is positioned to one side of the follicle, is surrounded by the fluid, called follicular fluid, in the follicle and by the granulosa cells. These are the cells that produce the female hormones, estrogen and progesterone. The granulosa cells also produce the substances that mature the egg and provide the energy for its growth. We do not yet know exactly how this happens. We do know that there are about five million or so granulosa cells in each follicle surrounding each egg. All these cells are there primarily for one purpose, that is to supply just one cell, the egg, with all its needs until after ovulation. This must be one of the few situations where so many cells serve only one other cell.

Most eggs remain in a 'primitive' stage, and never even have a follicle develop around them. Only those that do will be capable of going on to ovulation. Extraordinarily, there is huge wearing down of cells even at this stage, as far more follicles start to develop than ovulate. We think that follicular development starts about three months before ovulation and that this is the result of stimulation by the pituitary gland, possibly by FSH – although this is certainly not the whole story.

At the start of the menstrual cycle, FSH from the pituitary gland begins to stimulate more vigorously the Graafian follicles that have already started to develop. As the follicles swell in size, one follicle outstrips the others in growth. It is this follicle, called the dominant follicle, that will shed the egg in that cycle by ovulating. The other follicles will shrink in size and disappear altogether. Yet again, we have no definite idea how the body decides which follicle will ovulate in a given cycle, but it is this mechanism that prevents humans from having a litter, unlike many other animals. As the dominant follicle swells from the size of a pinhead to the size of a large grape, the granulosa cells pour out increasing quantities of the hormone estrogen. Estrogen prepares the uterus to grow, to receive any pregnancy that may be conceived. During the first ten days or so after menstruation, the level of the estrogen rises in the bloodstream. When a certain level is reached, this rising level is detected by the brain, which sends messages to the pituitary gland to slow down the production of FSH. Rising levels of estrogen also now appear to trigger the secretion of LH by the pituitary. The exact mechanism is also not fully understood, but we know that the message to the pituitary is an indirect one and is made by the hypothalamus. The hypothalamus is part of the brain, a short distance away from the pituitary. It is about the size of a bean. It also secretes hormones (called releasing hormones) that stimulate the pituitary to produce LH. We shall hear more about these hormones later (see Chapter 3) as they are now used in the treatment of certain types of infertility.

Once LH production is triggered, the amount produced rises rapidly. Increasing amounts of LH in the bloodstream are detected by the ovary and the final process of ovulation is set in motion. The follicle ruptures about thirty-six hours after the start of LH production by the pituitary. LH also has an important effect on the

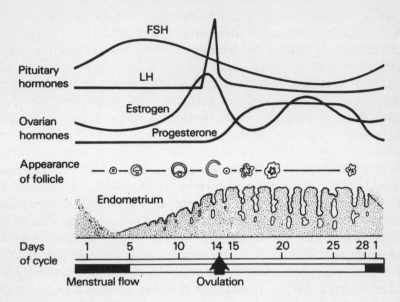

The menstrual cycle

granulosa cells in the follicle and remarkably converts them to a different chemical reaction. Although some estrogen is still produced, the granulosa cells now start to manufacture the hormone progesterone in steadily increasing amounts. The change in manufacture of hormones is accompanied by a change in appearance of the follicle. After ovulation it tends to fill with blood (this may be why some women get pain in the mid-cycle) and the granulosa cells turn a yellow-orange colour. Over the next few days, the follicle becomes increasingly yellow to become the corpus luteum, or yellow body. About ten days after ovulation, progesterone secretion by the corpus luteum virtually ceases (because the pituitary stops producing much LH) and about fourteen days after ovulation, the period starts.

Menstruation

Most women bleed every month. The exact length of time between each menstrual period depends partly on how often you ovulate. Normally, you would expect to bleed about fourteen days after ovulation. However, it is quite possible to have periods even when you are not ovulating. Although you may miss periods if you are not ovulating, this is not the only cause of absent periods; it may also be due to the uterus having certain abnormalities (see page 80).

Menstrual bleeding is the result of the shedding of the lining of the uterus. It occurs only in humans and some monkeys – just another little piece of evidence that shows we are closer to the apes than perhaps we like to think. Lower animals do not menstruate at all.

At the beginning of the menstrual cycle, when the period is just finishing, the lining of the uterus is very thin. If you read the section above on ovulation carefully enough, you will remember that before ovulation – which coincides with the first half of your menstrual cycle – one ovary is manufacturing increasing amounts of estrogen. This causes the uterus to enlarge imperceptibly. Estrogen also encourages the lining of the uterus to grow thicker. This thickening of the uterine lining, or endometrium to give it its proper name, is the beginning of preparing the uterus to receive an embryo – should you happily get pregnant in that cycle. Estrogen also stimulates the lining to grow little glands (see the diagram opposite). These glands, which are invisible to the naked eye, look like little pits on the surface of the lining if viewed under a microscope. These glands will later produce fluid, called uterine fluid, which helps to nourish sperms and embryos that may find their way into the uterus.

Once ovulation has taken place, the ovary produces progesterone, manufactured by the corpus luteum. Progesterone, too, has an important action on the uterus and stimulates the growth of many rich blood vessels which supply the endometrium. It also causes the little glands in the endometrium to grow bigger and gets them to produce the uterine fluid. About seven days after ovulation, progesterone manufacture is at a peak and the glands are working quite vigorously. This coincides with the time that an embryo would normally be expected to start to implant in the uterine cavity. The lining of the uterus is prepared to provide the ideal environment for an embryo to 'bed down' and develop attachments to the uterus. Once the embryo has started to implant in this way, it will begin to produce progesterone of its own, and this encourages further development of the uterine lining.

In most months, however, even entirely fertile women do not conceive, and within ten days of ovulation progesterone production starts to decrease. A rapid fall in the level of progesterone results in cessation of the growth stimulus to the uterine lining. The rich blood vessels contract and the lining of the uterus, which so recently grew thick, is starved of oxygen carried in those blood vessels. Loss of the blood supply leads to sudden death of the lining, which starts to break up and fragment. Thus the lining starts to be shed, together with some bleeding from the ends of the blood vessels. This is the beginning of the menstrual period.

Although we know a good deal about the growth and development of the endometrium, we know remarkably little about what happens to embryos inside the uterine cavity and precisely how they implant. We do know that there is less chance of satisfactory implantation if the embryo arrives too early in the uterus, before the endometrium is fully developed. It has even been suggested that this may be a cause for very early miscarriages. We also know that a pregnancy may be unlikely if the embryo arrives too late. We do not know exactly how an embryo implants and we certainly do not understand why so many apparently entirely healthy embryos never implant properly but are lost by the next menstrual period. Many people wonder where lost embryos, or indeed lost eggs, go if this part of the reproductive process doesn't work. The answer is that both the embryo and the egg are far smaller than the full stop at the end of this sentence. If they don't implant they just shrink away and are absorbed in the body or lost outside it, via the vagina.

Transport of eggs and sperms and the ovaries

Obviously, before you can get pregnant, the sperm and egg have to meet. This is a more difficult journey than you might expect. The story of how this happens is truly remarkable.

At intercourse, the average man ejaculates anything from one hundred million to eight hundred million sperms into the vagina. Many of these sperms immediately trickle out of the vagina. Most just remain inside the vagina, where they rapidly die because they are killed by the vagina's natural acidity. A small proportion, not more than a few million at most, find their way into the cervix or, more precisely, into the cervical mucus, which is the fluid in the cervix (see Chapter 6). Unless intercourse takes place within about a week before ovulation, virtually none of the sperm will survive because, either there will not be any mucus to speak of or the mucus will be thick (hostile) and impenetrable to sperm (see Chapter 6).

Once sperm have entered the mucus, the majority will stay put. The sperm in the mucus can be regarded as a reservoir. Over the next days, a few will swim up through the mucus and into the uterine cavity. This release of sperm from the mucus will continue regularly until the mucus becomes thick again (under the influence of progesterone after ovulation). This mechanism has an important biological function. The reservoir of sperm actually prevents the need for humans to have intercourse each time to get pregnant. This is different from most animals, who tend to have intercourse when they are on heat, the only time when many female animals are receptive to the male. The human mechanism allows people to make love when they feel like it.

Sperm in the uterus seem to be rapidly transported into the tubes. We have very little idea how this happens, but we think that the uterus itself continually contracts and expands and acts rather like a pump, forcing sperms onward. Some doctors believe that good sperm transport is more likely if the woman has an orgasm because that may encourage these muscular contractions. We do know for certain that orgasm is inessential to fertility and we also know that it by no means pushes all the sperm up into the tubes.

From the uterus, the sperms enter the tubes, where they seem to stay in another reservoir. This is in the part of the tubes closest to the uterus (see the diagram on page 14). This is not just a case of the sperm swimming to this point. The speed at which human sperm swim has been carefully measured; we know, if left to their own devices, it would take sperms about seven to eleven hours to swim the distance of the relatively long journey between cervix and uterus. In fact, sperm can be found in the fallopian tube within fifteen minutes of their being deposited in the vagina. This has actually been shown in volunteers undergoing operations on their fallopian tubes.

Once in the fallopian tube, sperms are capable of staying there for several days. This ensures that any egg entering the tube will be

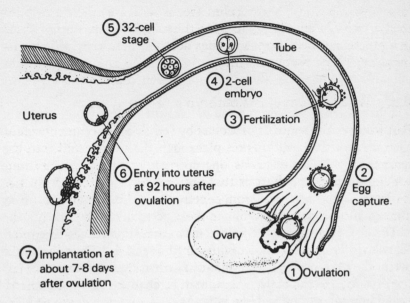

The fertilization of an egg, and implantation and growth of the embryo

potentially capable of being fertilized – even if a couple have not had intercourse for several days. This means *that careful timing of intercourse is almost certainly unnecessary for people to conceive.* Although most of the sperm stay in the part of the tube closest to the uterus, fertilization of the egg occurs in the outer end of the tube, near the ovary.

Not many people realize that each of us spent the first three or four days of life in the tube, not in the uterus. The fallopian tubes must be the most complicated pipes in the body. Not only does one of them pick up the egg from the ovary after ovulation, but it transports the egg in a carefully timed way to the site of fertilization. It has the unique ability of transporting the egg in one direction while simultaneously transporting sperms in the opposite direction. If the egg is fertilized and an embryo forms, then the tube is responsible for moving it into the uterus. It takes about ninety hours to do this, a period carefully timed so that the egg will arrive in the uterus when its lining is suitably receptive. The tube also supplies foodstuffs to the developing early embryo and removes waste products. These facts may seem of particular interest if you have a problem with the tubes (see Chapter 4). They help to explain why tubal surgery to open the tubes doesn't always result in a pregnancy, because the various delicate transport mechanisms may have been upset by scarring.

Early development of the embryo and implantation

Fertilization, the series of processes by which one sperm enters and then fuses with the egg, takes place in the outer end of the tube, near the ovary. As soon as one sperm enters the egg, the egg produces a chemical barrier that prevents any other sperm of the thousands surrounding it from penetrating it. This prevents certain abnormalities from developing in the embryo.

The fertilized egg now develops in the tube. Over the next twelve to twenty hours, the egg divides into two cells. Each of these divides into two and then again. These cell divisions occur at intervals of about fifteen hours, so that by the time ninety or so hours have elapsed (the time when the embryo enters the uterus) there are about sixty-four cells. In the early stages of development – say at around eight cells – each one has the potential to become a human being. This is of interest to people undergoing test-tube baby treatment. Even if seven of the eight cells in the embryo that is put back (see Chapter 10) are clearly dying, leaving only one good cell, there is still a chance of pregnancy and this pregnancy will be normal. Another interesting fact is that, of the sixty-four or so cells that enter the uterus, only a few of them – perhaps no more than eight – will make the baby. The rest of the embryo will go to form the placenta (afterbirth) and membranes that surround the developing foetus.

When the embryo enters the uterus, it may float around for two or three days, still growing. It does not stick to the lining of the uterus until about seven days after fertilization, when the process of implantation starts. At this stage (about which we know very little) the embryo begins burrowing into the lining of the uterus and the placenta starts to form. At this stage the embryo starts to produce pregnancy hormone (human chorionic gonadotrophin – HCG) and this can be detected by highly sensitive and expensive tests. These are not widely available and most women will have no idea at all that they are pregnant until at least seven days later, when the expected period is missed. It seems that implantation is a very fragile business – we know that at least 40 per cent of human embryos that enter the uterus do not implant but just die. This is one reason why even fertile people usually do not conceive immediately.

Many embryos are also lost after implantation, around the time of menstruation. Sometimes there may be a delay of a period for one or two days, followed by a normal bleed. This is also very common in both fertile and infertile women and is the earliest form of miscarriage (see Chapter 7). If you are infertile and occasionally have delayed periods in cycles in which you definitely ovulated, you may well be getting pregnant. It is worth finding out whether you can get one of the sensitive early pregnancy tests done, because it is very reassuring to know that you are capable of conceiving after some tubal surgery, for example.

At about fourteen days, the embryo has implanted firmly. Although it can still miscarry, the chance is less likely now. At this stage the first organs start to form – the nervous system begins at about fifteen to sixteen days and the heart a little later. Fourteen days is the latest stage when an embryo can split into two to form twins.

MYTHS AND LEGENDS ABOUT INFERTILITY

Throughout this book, I have tried to expose what I believe to be mythology. Because infertility is so common and because it affects us in a very personal and private way, a huge number of myths have been built up. I regret to say that some of these myths are perpetuated by experts and even by writers of books! They are harmful, because they give a false impression. Here are some of the myths that I am confronted with most often.

Pregnancy always happens if you have sex at the right time

Quite untrue. It takes the average fertile couple five months to conceive normally, even when they have sex very regularly. It may take even longer. Only about 15 per cent of people conceive in the first cycle of regular intercourse.

We must time intercourse carefully if we have a fertility problem

Generally speaking, this is also untrue. Careful timing of inter-course often does more harm than good. If the woman has normal mucus in the cervix, then she has a reservoir of sperm that will last for at least three days – possibly longer. Sex two or three times a week is enough. If you time sex rigorously you may almost certainly end up under strain and both of you will suffer. Things get worse if one of you doesn't feel like making love or if work has taken one of you away from home.

Timing can also be a mistake because it is very easy to misjudge the fertile time. Perfectly normal women do not always ovulate on the fourteenth day. Ovulation can occur occasionally on the seventh or twenty-third day of the cycle, for example. Temperature charting will not reveal this until afterwards; this is why I am generally opposed to anyone keeping temperature charts for longer than about three months.

I believe that the strain involved in continually trying to find the right time may actually prevent pregnancy. I have seen evidence of this in women coming to my clinic.

I'm not getting pregnant because all the sperm run out after intercourse

Untrue. All women lose semen from the vagina after sex. This is normal and depends on the volume of the semen ejaculated. The more discharge, the more sperm were there to start with. Enough sperm will get to the cervix, from where they don't escape (see Chapter 6).

I need to lie on my stomach after sex

There are many variations on this one. There is not the slightest evidence that any particular position is more likely to help conception. This applies to positions both during and after intercourse. Adopt an interesting position if it's fun, but not to get pregnant.

My uterus is tilted backwards (retroverted) and this is stopping conception

This is discussed in Chapter 5. Quite simply, about one in four fertile women have a uterus that is tilted in some way. Any form of trouble is rare.

Ovulation occurs from alternate ovaries in alternate months

Not so. People who have only one tube or one ovary frequently ask about this. Which ovary ovulates in a given month is entirely random. We cannot predict which one will ovulate until about the eighth day of the cycle, when ultrasound measurements generally show that one follicle is larger than others. However, if you have only one ovary, you will usually ovulate every month from that side (see Chapter 3).

Some women have only one functioning tube. We know that it is possible for the tube to collect an egg that has come from either side; however, we think that the tube is more likely most times to pick up eggs from the ovary next to it rather than from the opposite side.

If you're having periods, you're ovulating

Not necessarily (see Chapter 3). Regular periods do not guarantee ovulation, although if your periods are absolutely regular it is more likely to be taking place.

Not having periods is bad for my body

Some infertile women have very scanty periods or no periods at all. Some treatments for infertility (like those for endometriosis – see Chapter 4) may involve drugs that stop your periods for several months. Many people think that if you don't menstruate regularly, waste products or poisons are building up in the body. This is quite untrue. It will not affect your health at all if your periods have stopped. However, if you are having no periods, it is worth consulting your family doctor because there may be an underlying cause that needs some treatment.

Frigidity causes infertility

Untrue. There is no evidence that failure to be aroused during sex makes a significant difference to fertility. It is possible that a good orgasm may help with sperm transport or even ovulation, but there is no evidence that not having an orgasm prevents pregnancy.

Having sex too frequently weakens the sperm

Almost certainly not true. The only evidence that I know of on this subject shows that the more often you have sex, the more likely you are to conceive. This certainly does not suggest that the sperm count is weakened by a great deal of sexual activity.

Even if a man has a low sperm count, there is very little evidence to show that by saving it all up and having sex less frequently there will be a better chance of pregnancy. However, there is some evidence which shows that some men may improve their sperm count by having sex more frequently.

Infertile men are weaklings

A total lie. Some infertile men make the best lovers, just as some infertile women are very good in bed. We confuse sexuality and fertility in our minds but they are quite different. Male infertility in no way reflects on any other aspect of a man's potency, strength or masculinity.

Infertility is caused by the woman

Yes, but only half the time! Careful investigation has shown that although women are slightly more likely to have a fertility problem than men, 30 per cent of infertility is caused by the man alone. In another 20 per cent, the man and woman both contribute to the partnership's infertility.

Test-tube baby treatment is likely to solve my problem

This is not true. Test-tube baby treatment (see Chapter 10) is generally the *least successful of all infertility treatments* and is mostly the last resort. Please, before considering test-tube baby treatment, make certain that you have been fully and carefully investigated and that you have had the appropriate treatment. Unfortunately, there is a tendency for infertile men and women to receive treatment before proper testing has been done and before the cause of infertility, the diagnosis, has been clearly established. Because infertility causes desperation, people frequently seek test-tube baby treatment when a much simpler treatment would carry a better chance of success.

Which doctor should I go to?

In Britain or Australia, you should go initially to your general practitioner. He or she may do some simple tests first, such as sperm counts, before deciding whether you need a more specialized opinion. Some general practitioners are extremely interested in infertility and will actively start investigations. Others may recommend referral directly to a hospital. It is worth both of you going to see the specialist together – usually a gynaecologist – for your first appointment so that you can give each other a bit of support; such an appointment often causes considerable nerves. At moments like this it is worth remembering that it is very common for both members of a partnership to contribute towards infertility.

If you live in the United States, it is quite usual to go to somebody more expert without first seeing a general or family physician. Seek a specialist who deals in infertility if possible, rather than a doctor who practises general gynaecology.

In general in the UK, you are safer at least initially going under the National Health Service. Unfortunately, it is fair to say that NHS infertility treatment is rather uneven and some units are less interested or less able to cope with these problems than others. If you find that your local NHS hospital is not able to provide detailed care, you should ask for a referral to a major NHS centre. On the whole this is usually a better bet than going privately. People often think that if they pay, they will have access to better treatment. Regrettably this is not always true. Of course, there are many excellent people offering private infertility treatment. However, in my experience, private treatment is quite frequently very poor and also expensive. My advice is to be wary of going for private treatment simply because you may feel more comfortable in pleasant surroundings or because a good NHS unit has told you there is nothing to be done.

Having warned you about the risks of private treatment, there is still nothing to prevent your taking a good second opinion. Indeed, that is your entitlement and you shouldn't feel embarrassed about asking for this. If you do decide to go privately, there are certain questions you should ask yourself. In many ways these same questions apply also to NHS practitioners. The questions are:

- Am I really being investigated thoroughly and are all the tests being looked at personally by my doctor?
- Am I being offered treatment, for example clomiphene, tubal surgery or IVF, before a diagnosis has been firmly established?
- Is the clinic I am attending able to offer all treatments or is it interested primarily in offering one treatment, for example, test-tube baby treatment?
- Are the success rates I am being quoted those attained by the doctor I am talking to, or are they results quoted in general and attained by others?
- Do I feel comfortable with the doctor with whom I am discussing my problem?
- Does the private doctor I am seeing also see NHS patients as a consultant in a general hospital? (Having a consultant appointment in the state system is a yardstick of competence.)
- In the UK or Australia: if my gynaecologist does not hold a consultant appointment, does he or she have a higher qualification, such as the MRCOG or FRCOG?
- If in the US, is my doctor Board Certified in the subspeciality of endocrinology and infertility?
- Shall I be given a detailed written report of what has been done?

If the answer to any of these questions is no, you should at least think carefully about the advice and treatment you may be buying. In later chapters you will see the complexity of causes, and the necessity for the best help. First I describe some of the immediate problems couples have who are faced with infertility.

2

The experience of infertility

WHAT DOES IT FEEL LIKE TO BE INFERTILE?

What effect does infertility have on your self-esteem? How do you cope with friendships and social contacts? How do you protect yourself against repeated disappointments and intrusive treatments? What do other people do about it?

In their book, *Coping with Childlessness* (see page 190), Diane and Peter Houghton point out that the experience and reaction to infertility varies greatly from person to person. This is an important point. Nevertheless, most infertile people go through certain emotions and the feelings that they express tend to fall into a pattern. In this chapter, I try to outline how people often feel. These emotions are frequently very strong indeed and it is not surprising that it is widely believed that the emotional turmoil some people suffer may actually make it more difficult to conceive. In the second half of the chapter, I try to evaluate whether there is such a condition as psychological infertility.

Early worries

Most people do not get terribly worried if they fail to conceive during the first few months of a partnership. The gradual realization that there may be a problem is something that couples tend to shrug off to start with. Very often it is the woman who takes the initiative by going to see her doctor, sometimes without her partner being fully aware of her worry. It is also quite common for her man to appear unconcerned or indifferent, which can mask a gnawing doubt. Some couples go several years before seeking medical help.

Disbelief

The first real shock of infertility often comes when a couple see friends starting their family without trouble. The reality of their own situation is hard to believe and they are likely to deny that they genuinely have a problem. Very often infertile people become increasingly anxious and restless. Fear is common and the first visit to a specialist can be much more traumatic than the doctor appears to realize.

Anger, guilt and frustration

Infertility produces bursts of anger, which may be directed towards one's spouse, the doctor, the clinic or the tests that seem to give dubious results. Infertile couples can feel most frustrated when a complicated test such as a laparoscopy (see Chapter 3) fails to find an abnormality. Although discovering something definitely wrong may mean that the chances of a pregnancy are not good, some people appear to be more frustrated if the findings at laparoscopy are normal. Anger is also directed at oneself and this produces feelings of guilt – the feeling that you have brought your infertility upon yourself is almost always experienced at some stage. Another emotion that you are likely to have is resentment that others do not seem to understand how you feel. You may also be bitterly unhappy at losing control – at having to rely on a doctor to help with what should happen naturally. Anger may be felt, too, at people who have children, at having to wait in a clinic where there may also be pregnant women waiting for antenatal appointments and, particularly, at women who are undergoing termination of pregnancy.

Depression and feelings of pointlessness

Nearly all infertile women experience depression at some stage or another. It develops gradually and may become most acute just before or just after your period – especially if the period is delayed for some reason.

Depression may just make you feel very sad or tearful. You may actually have had periods of sleeplessness, loss of appetite, or other body disturbances such as constipation. Depression can be accompanied by the feeling that things are not worth enjoying, that it is not worth trying to be successful in your job – because you have no children to appreciate the material advantages you may be able to produce in life. You may come to think that there is no point in going to normal social engagements, parties or meetings any more. Depression makes people withdraw into themselves, avoid friendships and refuse to share their feelings. Isolation is a common expression of infertility, and it often comes as a surprise to infertile couples that others have had exactly the same feelings.

Along with depression can go a loss of self-esteem. Both partners feel as if they are failures. For a man, infertility may first present a problem just when he is trying hard to develop a career. If his job is not going well, he may feel particularly worthless as a 'double failure' in life.

Problems with sex

Most couples find that at some stage their sexual relationship is affected by infertility. Often it's just that making love ceases being spontaneous and becomes planned and cold. Pleasure may be a thing of the past and many women stop having orgasms. Men may experience impotence or premature ejaculation. Very often, the need to have sex produces strong feelings of anxiety. So many women explain that there 'seems no point in sex any more – my body can't respond and is just useless'. It is common, too, to feel unattractive or unloved and many couples find that they end up having sex at increasingly infrequent intervals. Unfortunately, some doctors appear to show little understanding of these problems and their advice to have intercourse at 'precisely the right time' or suggestion of help with a post-coital test may make matters seem much worse.

Grief and bereavement

Persistent infertility leads to grief. The hopelessness of the situation can lead to obsession – perhaps the desire to chase every possible option or treatment, no matter how illogical. Quite frequently, grieving couples seek repeated second opinions, when an earlier one fails to provide relief.

Many of the feelings of grief are a reaction to the inability to give life. People who lose a parent or a friend are usually supported in their bereavement, but infertile couples often feel that they have no one to turn to, no support to lean on. Parents may refuse to accept the situation, and it can be very difficult to explain to them how you feel. Friends who have children may appear embarrassed or unfeeling, and they fail to appreciate the anger and frustration you live with every day.

Grief may have positive advantages in the end. If you are absolutely infertile, the process of grief, bereavement and mourning may lead to a final healing. This can resolve what is otherwise an entirely destructive situation.

In the remainder of this chapter, I explore whether some of the feelings I have just described could actually cause the infertility. At various points in the rest of the book, I examine the ways you may come to terms with some of them. Chapter 13, 'Ten points for infertile couples', is written partly to show how you can protect yourself from the more corrosive aspects of infertility and infertility treatments.

PSYCHOLOGICAL INFERTILITY

At some stage or another nearly all infertile couples wonder whether their tangled emotions are causing the infertility. If you have been trying harder and harder for a long time and there is still no obvious cause for your childlessness, inevitably you begin to think your anxiety is itself the problem. One of the difficulties is the vicious circle you are in. The harder and longer you try, the more disturbed you feel. The question is, is there any real evidence that your emotions are preventing you from conceiving?

The case against psychological infertility

I find it difficult to believe that emotional turmoil alone is an important cause of infertility. If it were true, you would expect people under exceptional stress not to get pregnant. This does not seem to be the case. Take the example of the young girl having sex with her boyfriend and not using contraception. She may be desperately worried that she might get pregnant, so much so that it causes enormous stress in her sexual relationship. This never seems to reduce the disasters that we see, and the frightened requests for secret abortions. To look at another example, think of the women who suffer the trauma of rape, with the most horrific stress. Yet statistics show that the chances of getting pregnant after a single act of rape are actually higher than the chances of conceiving from a single episode of intercourse in a loving relationship. Why this should be is not clear, but it certainly doesn't support the idea that infertility is caused by extreme stress. If this were a serious bar to conception, you would also expect that women suffering great hardship would not conceive readily. Yet unwanted pregnancy is very common in populations where the most severe privation is normal – psychological infertility doesn't seem to be a problem in famine-struck Asia, for example. Finally, think of couples undergoing test-tube baby treatment. By the time an embryo is transferred, the woman is often severely stressed and some women are much more emotional than others. Their attitude and emotional state seem to have remarkably little effect on the chance of conception.

The case for psychological infertility

Having considered why emotions don't seem to make much difference, let us look at the other side of the coin. What evidence is there for emotionally induced infertility?

Many animals in zoos, even when well fed and well treated, are much less fertile than when they are in the wild. Zoos worldwide have always had difficulty, for example, trying to breed giant pandas. Most research workers know that one of the most fertile creatures, the rabbit, is bred with difficulty if there is a great deal of noise in the animal house where the rabbits are kept. I remember how difficult it used to be to breed rabbits in our own animal house when a new technician, a stranger, was first employed to look after them. They started to breed again only when they were used to him. This is certainly evidence for psychological factors preventing normal fertility. Humans may also be like this. It is well known that women in prison or women who were brutally kept in concentration camps had severe disturbances of their periods and often did not ovulate.

Perhaps one of the most often quoted cases of psychological infertility are those couples who, after years of tension trying hard for a baby, finally adopt. Within weeks of the adoption, they conceive naturally without any medical help. It is difficult to prove whether this is just due to chance.

Ellen and her husband, Paul, had been trying for a baby for six years. Extensive tests did not show an obvious cause for infertility. Ellen had never had children, though Paul had had a child by another woman many years earlier. In spite of this, Paul's tests were not entirely normal and I thought it was almost certain that he was the cause of the problem. I continued to treat them both, but five more years passed without pregnancy.

One day Ellen came to see me by herself. We were both feeling depressed about her problem and I said I felt she would just have to accept that Paul's sperm count was low and had not improved. At this point Ellen broke down and said she had been hiding something from everybody. She said she was sure the fertility problem was hers because for years she had simultaneously been trying to get pregnant by her boyfriend, Simon. Simon was married and fertile with three young children. Paul knew nothing of this relationship. 'Now, you see, it must be my fault, but I don't know how to reassure Paul, who feels so guilty,' she said.

I saw a very unhappy Ellen for six more months. At the back of my mind I felt that she ought to resolve her trouble by making a definite break – we discussed various possibilities, including her getting divorced. She said she desperately wanted to marry

Simon and he had told her he would divorce his wife. One day Ellen came to the clinic, deeply upset.

'It's all over – Simon and his wife are emigrating. He's going to work in California and I've told Paul everything. Now I'll never have a baby.'

I gently suggested that perhaps this was all for the best.

Seven weeks later Ellen returned to my clinic with a positive pregnancy test.

This kind of story is not unusual in infertility clinics. The speed that people get pregnant when an emotional situation like Ellen's is resolved makes one feel that perhaps, after all, we are sometimes the cause of our own problems.

What other pressures are there on infertile couples that might make things worse?

Family and friends

For some couples, the biggest problem is parents. Although they may show considerable sympathy for you when they finally come to terms with your infertility, some parents feel very aggrieved at first and deprived at the thought that there will be no grand-children. They may put you under unspoken pressure by never raising the subject; or they may press you by suggesting what you should do about treatment when you have already taken certain decisions. Very frequently, there is more than a hint of criticism. Your parents-in-law are liable to think it is your fault, even if the cause is not known, and the message you feel you are getting is that you are an inadequate spouse for their child. Your parents' affection for grandchildren by one of your brothers or sisters and their obvious satisfaction at a new pregnancy may be particularly painful. Sisters can be a threat, too, and it is remarkably common for infertile women to find it impossible to spend time in a brother's or sister's house, especially if it is full of young children.

Another pressure may be the attitude of friends. Even your closest friends may try to protect you by refusing to bring up the subject of children. This reinforces the guilt and inadequacy you feel about being infertile. Although you feel quite unable to mention the subject yourself, the conspiracy of silence only increases your lack of self-esteem. A dinner party with people you know only slightly may be a huge hardship. It is surprising how often the subject of children crops up followed by stifled embarrassment from those who simply wish to protect you.

Sex

Few fertile people are aware of the stress that infertility causes in your sexual relationship. Sex may stop being enjoyable when you feel you must have intercourse at the 'right time'. Loss of desire is a frequent by-product of infertility. Perhaps this itself increases the infertility and some specialists even think that loss of orgasm for the woman can decrease fertility. Whether pleasurable intercourse improves the chance of conception is not clear, but it might be better for you to try to have sex only when you really feel like it, even though you think you may be missing the time around ovulation. One or two nights of pleasure may be better than daily attempts and frustration.

Anxiety, holidays and giving up work

Your specialist may encourage you to get out of your domestic environment a bit more often. Weekends away, short holidays and even an afternoon's walk together in a pleasant park nearby may be invaluable if things are getting on top of you. Apart from anything else, relaxing together regularly should help to break the tension between you and allow you to communicate better. It should help improve any strain over sex as well as the other pent-up thoughts about the infertility. Some women have also found giving up their job has been most therapeutic. Not surprisingly, others find that starting a new job is of great benefit!

Our present feeling is that the evidence for your emotional state being a real cause for infertility is sketchy. It is true it may contribute, but probably only to a tiny degree. To be aware of this problem and to meet it sensibly is an important part of your battle, not only to improve your chances, but also to help you stand up to the long periods of uncertainty and come out feeling ready to try another time.

3

Trouble with ovulation

Every woman fails to ovulate during her monthly cycle from time to time. Some women always ovulate irregularly. Infertility is likely only if you don't ovulate frequently. About 30 per cent of infertile couples cannot have a baby because the woman doesn't ovulate. Fortunately, though, in over 90 per cent of cases we are able to stimulate ovulation successfully using drugs. Although this may be the most frequent cause of infertility, it is also the one with the best chances of successful treatment.

WHAT ARE THE CAUSES OF FAILURE OF OVULATION?

There are three basic reasons why you may not ovulate:

1. There is a hormonal or chemical problem somewhere in your body. This is the cause for 70 per cent of women not ovulating.
2. There is a functional problem, meaning simply that although there is no major change, your ovaries don't work in a particular cycle. This can happen if, for example, you are emotionally upset. It is the cause in between 10 and 15 per cent of women with ovulation failure.
3. The ovaries are physically damaged, abnormal from birth or absent, or they just do not contain any eggs. This is probably the reason in 10 to 15 per cent of cases.

Hormonal and chemical problems

- About half the women with hormonal or chemical problems do not produce enough follicles for the egg to develop (see Chapter 1). This may be due to lack of hormones from the pituitary gland or the hypothalamus, or to a problem in the ovaries themselves.
- There may be a problem with the pituitary gland (about 10 per cent of women with ovulation failure). The pituitary gland is the 'master' gland (see page 6) which controls most other hormone glands in the body. It is extremely powerful and if it stops working normally, this can affect the function of other glands under its control, including the ovary. The breast is also partly under the control of the pituitary, and it can affect the production of breast milk.
- There is a problem with the hypothalamus (about 10 per cent of cases); this is the part of the brain that controls the pituitary (see page 9). Changes in the chemical messages produced in the hypothalamus can greatly affect the pituitary, and therefore the ovaries.
- There are other unrelated hormone problems (perhaps 5 per cent of all cases), for example, a thyroid disorder. Women with overactive or underactive thyroid glands sometimes fail to ovulate.

Functional problems

- There are, of course, many occasions when you may not ovulate normally. Girls generally don't ovulate regularly until their menstrual cycle is properly established, in their late teens. Towards the end of reproductive life – that is, in the late thirties and early forties – you will also ovulate less often. This is usually the first function to stop at the time near the menopause, long before your periods finally finish.

  Women who have taken the contraceptive pill often worry that their ovulation may be affected afterwards, especially if they don't have normal periods on stopping the pill. There is no real evidence that the pill is responsible for failure to ovulate. If your periods have stopped, this should be exceptionally easy to put right with the drugs described later in this chapter.

- The ovaries stop working completely. Only about 5 per cent of women don't ovulate for this reason. The ovary may sometimes contain no eggs and just cannot respond to drugs. Complete ovarian failure in a woman of childbearing age is a rare cause of infertility. Very occasionally, ovaries that seem to have failed completely may suddenly start working again and produce eggs. The reason for this happy event is not understood.

  If you begin having more frequent periods after you've been told that this is your problem, it may be a sign that you have started ovulating again (see below). However, this is certainly not necessarily true and it is easy to have your hopes raised falsely. Talk to your doctor by all means, and be guided by his or her opinion.

- A serious emotional upset – such as bad depression, imprisonment or a severe shock – can so upset the chemistry of your brain temporarily that the hypothalamus stops working to full capacity. This is not nearly as common as infertile couples tend to believe, and the psychological disturbance usually has to be very traumatic. Mere worry alone does not normally cause you to stop ovulating (see also Chapter 1).

- You may ovulate but the follicle containing the egg does not burst, so the process stops right at the beginning. Alternatively, the follicle may burst but no egg escapes.

- The ovaries are physically damaged, or sometimes many small cysts form inside them, preventing them from working properly. This is known as polycystic ovarian disease (see page 50).

IS FAILURE TO OVULATE YOUR PROBLEM?

How can you tell whether you are ovulating? There are a number of signs that suggest whether you are or not, although these do not amount to cast-iron proof. At least they will give you an indication, which you can discuss with your doctor. If you are ovulating you are more likely to have:

Absolutely regular periods If your cycle is more or less regular every twenty-six to twenty-nine days and never varies by more than one or two days, it is most likely that you are ovulating.

Breast tenderness and painful periods You may get sore or 'full' breasts in the cycles when you ovulate. This discomfort is greatest just before your period; some women who always ovulate get it quite badly.

Dull discomfort in the pelvis or lower back immediately before your period – called congestive dysmenorrhoea – tends also to happen more if you ovulate.

These feelings are not absolute proof but they are, in a funny sense, encouraging. Still, many perfectly ovulating women experience no breast or pelvic discomfort.

Pain in the middle of the cycle About 30 per cent of women feel mild or marked discomfort around the time of ovulation. This pain, which is sometimes called *Mittelschmertz* (the German for middle pain), is usually felt to one side of your abdomen, near the ovary that is ovulating. You may get this pain for a few hours once a month, almost exactly fourteen days before you start a period. The pain rarely lasts more than thirty-six hours.

A colourless discharge At the time of ovulation, your cervix becomes very active and produces a great deal of watery mucus. This is often enough to be noticed as a colourless or white discharge and can be sufficient to mark underclothing. It usually lasts not more than two days and is most noticeable about fifteen days before your period. This discharge may be bloodstained just at the time of ovulation, but this is less common.

You are unlikely to confuse this sort of bloodstain with bleeding. But if you do have heavy or persistent bleeding between periods you should talk to your doctor about it, as it can be a symptom of something more serious.

Signs that tend to indicate you are not ovulating are:

Your periods may stop totally   This is called amenorrhoea, and happens to about 20 per cent of women with ovulation problems – and of course when you are pregnant! This is not a definite signal of ovulation failure, though. Some women with amenorrhoea do ovulate.

Your periods may become infrequent or very scanty   This happens to another 40 per cent of women who are not ovulating. It is called oligomenorrhoea, and describes periods coming at intervals longer than every forty-two days.

Many women get very alarmed when they keep missing periods. But this doesn't necessarily mean you are starting the menopause or have a serious disease. The great majority of women with amenorrhoea and oligomenorrhoea are infertile and just not ovulating. In most cases this is due to the condition polycystic ovaries (see page 50), which is usually easily treated with tablets.

Infrequent periods are sometimes connected with changes in body weight; if you have gained or lost a great deal of weight recently this may be associated with your infrequent periods, and you may not be ovulating.

Your periods may be irregular   Many women who are infertile have irregular cycles, some of which occur at roughly twenty-eight day intervals, and others of up to forty or so days. This may mean you are not ovulating.

Lack of breast tenderness or pain   Although your periods are regular, you may not get breast tenderness or pain before menstruation. This is true of about 20 per cent of women who don't ovulate. If your periods are fairly regular you could be producing an egg but not enough of the hormone progesterone to help uterine development after ovulation (see page 10). This means that the egg may not survive; this is categorized as an ovulatory problem. This so-called luteal defect is now easier to treat, because we understand the mechanism of ovulation better.

You have noticed an increase in body or facial hair recently   This is quite likely also to be due to polycystic ovaries. As you will see later, it is usually fairly easily treated.

Making a temperature chart

If you suspect that you are not ovulating you can start by making a few simple tests yourself, before you speak to your doctor. One of the most popular ways of detecting ovulation is to keep a record of the changes in your temperature. A temperature chart is not a totally reliable way of confirming that you are ovulating but it can be useful, providing you don't get too depressed or emotional about it (see page 17).

Usually the body temperature drops immediately before ovulation and rises immediately afterwards. It then stays up until the period starts (see the diagrams on pages 36 and 37). This temperature rise is caused by the release of progesterone, which is produced by your ovary after ovulation. However, a lot of normally ovulating women produce high quantities of progesterone and yet their temperature does not rise, so charting is not infallible. If you want to try charting your own temperature, use a standard clinical thermometer, which you can buy from a chemist or drug store. You will also need a chart like the one in the diagram. This you can buy at the chemist, or you might pencil your temperature in on the chart here. The following points are important when temperature recording:

- Always keep the thermometer, along with your chart, beside your bed.
- Take your temperature, with the thermometer under your tongue, for two minutes, first thing before getting out of bed every morning. You should do this before drinking your first cup of tea or coffee, eating anything or smoking a cigarette.
- Read the thermometer immediately by finding where the mercury reaches and note the temperature marked on the side of the glass. Record your temperature straight away on your chart. Rinse the thermometer and shake it down to zero ready for the next day.
- It is a good idea to mark other relevant events on your chart. This could include any vaginal discharge, pelvic pain or

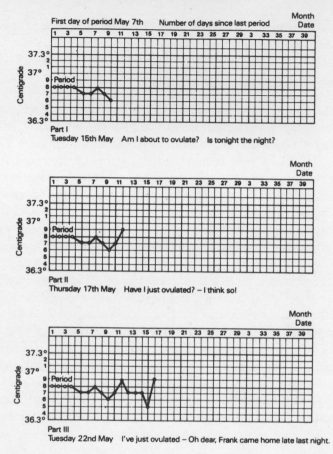

First day of period May 7th   Number of days since last period   Month Date

Part I
Tuesday 15th May   Am I about to ovulate?   Is tonight the night?

Part II
Thursday 17th May   Have I just ovulated? – I think so!

Part III
Tuesday 22nd May   I've just ovulated – Oh dear, Frank came home late last night.

The fallacy of the temperature record

bleeding between the periods. If you like, mark the days when you have intercourse. This means that later in the cycle you may be able to see if you had sex roughly at the right time of the month.

- If you have a sore throat or don't feel well, write this in on the chart too. Obviously, this may explain an abnormally high temperature.

Temperature charting has its pitfalls. Many normal women may not have a temperature rise after ovulation. Your record may remain flat even if ovulation is perfectly satisfactory. On the other

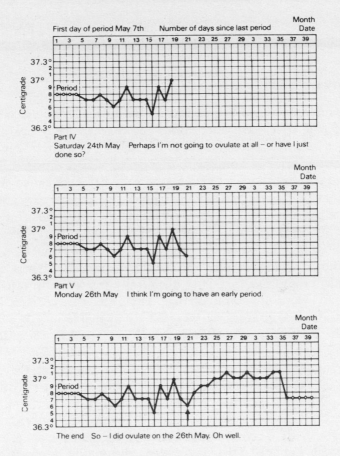

First day of period May 7th   Number of days since last period

Part IV
Saturday 24th May   Perhaps I'm not going to ovulate at all – or have I just done so?

Part V
Monday 26th May   I think I'm going to have an early period.

The end   So – I did ovulate on the 26th May. Oh well.

hand, some women have a rise in temperature in the second half of their cycle when an egg has not been shed. The biggest disadvantage is that taking your temperature every day continually reminds you of your fertility problem. You will be always trying to detect the initial temperature drop before ovulation. This can put pressure on you and your partner to make love so as not to miss the chance to conceive, while you or he may not feel in the least like having sex. This can cause terrible strain between partners. It can be dangerous and also futile, *because the temperature record is a poor predictor of imminent ovulation* and the supposed drop is more often than not irrelevant. Your temperature record is valuable really only at the end of a cycle when you or your doctor can look back and see how the record changed.

Urinary dip-stick

Fairly recently, a number of kits aimed to help you detect your most fertile time have come onto the market. They are manufactured by various companies, and nearly all of them involve you testing your urine at home with a paper or plastic dipstick. These kits are sold by chemists shops, and they use a so-called monoclonal antibody test for LH hormone. The kits are designed to detect when levels of LH in the blood, and therefore the urine, start to rise. As described in Chapter 1, LH rises about thirty-six hours before ovulation. Makers of the kits recommend that you time intercourse, having sex on the day of ovulation. The test is simple and usually involves dipping a chemically-treated strip into your urine and assessing a colour change. These kits were initiated in the United States, but are now increasingly available in other countries. In Britain, they cost from about £24 to £35 for just one month's supply.

I am not at all happy about these kits. For one thing, they have nearly all the disadvantages of temperature charting – with the added problem of expense! Their marketing has been accompanied by very considerable advertising and exaggerated claims for them have been made. Their commercial success depends to some extent on several 'medical' fallacies, and partly on the desperation of infertile women.

The first fallacy is that it is necessary to have intercourse on the day of ovulation to get pregnant. There is no proof that this is necessary. Certainly, as I mention elsewhere, precise timing of intercourse month after month can be emotionally demanding and damaging. Other fallacies are that the LH rise detected by these kits is followed by ovulation; also usage of these tests assumes that all women only have one rise in LH each month. Both these statements are certainly untrue. Moreover, kits are not always easy to use and several of my own friends or patients have found them to be unreliable or difficult to interpret. Most important, if you are one of many women who have an ovulation abnormality – especially if the levels of LH you are producing are higher than average (a common problem with polycystic ovaries, for example) – these hormone tests may give false readings. Consequently, although the advertising copy is very persuasive, these kits are best avoided. Apart from the emotional demands they make on you and their expense, there is absolutely no evidence at present that they help infertile women to conceive.

TESTS GIVEN BY YOUR DOCTOR

If you have already spoken to your doctor about your worries, there are a number of tests for ovulation you may be given that are much more conclusive than the temperature record.

These are the tests you are most likely to be offered. The order in which they are done will vary depending upon your circumstances and your doctor's decision. The order is not important; what is essential is that you have a full investigation. And this applies to all causes of infertility. Bear in mind that the results of two different tests can give conflicting answers, so your doctor's advice is important.

Blood progesterone measurement

A good way of detecting ovulation is to measure the amount of progesterone in the bloodstream. This starts rising a few hours before ovulation and peaks about seven days after ovulation. Just before your period, the level of progesterone falls quickly. Actually, it is this sudden drop in progesterone that causes your period, as the endometrium stops growing and dies when progesterone decreases (see page 11). If you get pregnant, you don't have a period because the pregnancy itself produces sufficient progesterone to maintain endometrial growth.

Blood progesterone measurements (or plasma progesterone measurements as they are usually called) are a pretty good way of seeing if ovulation takes place. They are not totally reliable for the same reasons as temperature charting: the ovary sometimes makes quite large amounts of progesterone without an egg actually leaving the ovary; also, ovulation may take place without progesterone rising very much. It is thought that this can even be a cause

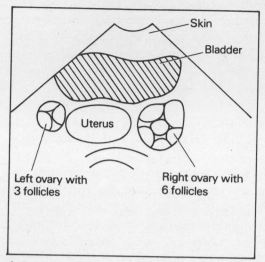

An ultrasound test showing follicles developing during treatment with fertility drugs

of infertility, and is sometimes called a defective luteal phase. The endometrium does not become secretory and so is not receptive to an embryo entering the uterus (see also below). Plasma progesterone levels can help in diagnosing this condition if several measurements are taken over five or six days. You may have to give a blood sample at the outpatient clinic each day. Unfortunately, progesterone tests are not cheap and they often need to be repeated.

Prolactin measurement

The prolactin, (the milk hormone), in your blood may be measured at the same time to ensure that you are not making too much of it. This can occasionally prevent you ovulating.

The test may also be done at any other time during your cycle.

Other hormone tests

Estrogen, luteinizing hormone (LH) and follicle stimulating hormone (FSH) all rise immediately before ovulation. They are highest about twenty-four hours before the egg leaves the ovary. Repeated testing of these hormones can help pinpoint ovulation very accurately, but as many tests may be needed these are not often used. Detailed hormone studies are reserved for women whose ovarian problems have not been diagnosed by the other methods.

Ultrasound

This is now used to check ovulation in some centres. The ultrasound machine is well known to pregnant women, as most expectant mothers will have at least one or two ultrasound tests during pregnancy to measure the size of the baby's head. Ultrasound, which is exactly like sonar used by ships to detect objects under the sea, gives an echo picture of the organs inside your body.

To check ovulation, echoes from the pelvic organs are taken. A fairly sophisticated machine and a skilful operator can detect the grape-like ovarian follicles (see Chapter 1). The follicle collapsing or filling with blood can also be detected using ultrasound. The difficulty with this test is that if the ovary is stuck to the bowel the echoes can be difficult to detect. Tubes filled with fluid (hydrosalpinx, see page 64) or an ovarian cyst can also make diagnosis difficult because the echoes from these look very similar to follicles. So the main problem with ultrasound is that the interpretation of the picture is still rather specialized. Most hospitals still do not have enough experienced people or sufficiently refined equipment.

The only disadvantage for you is that you need to have a full bladder for ultrasound tests, as the sound waves travel best through water. If your bladder is not absolutely full, the ovaries may not be detectable. Drinking large quantities of fluid – unfortunately usually water in most hospitals – to fill the bladder is rather uncomfortable. Other than that, it is a painless test.

Inspection of the cervix

Some doctors examine the cervix and its mucus at ovulation. If the mucus is very watery and copious and the cervix is slightly open, this may mean that ovulation is imminent. It is not a very accurate test but is sometimes useful when done with others (see also Chapter 6).

Endometrial biopsy

Many people will be familiar with endometrial biopsy (or EB as it is sometimes called). This involves taking a small scrap of the lining of the uterus, or endometrium, a few days before your period is due. The idea is quite simple: after ovulation the endometrium gets ready to receive any embryo that may enter the uterine cavity (see page 11). This change is caused by increased production of progesterone. Most women make enough progesterone to cause these secretory changes only after ovulation. If ovulation does not take place, not enough progesterone is made, and the endometrium does not get ready to receive an embryo.

It is quite simple to take a small piece (or biopsy) of the endometrium, stain it and examine it under a microscope. Your doctor may do this by inserting a small tube through the cervix that will scrape or suck the side of the uterine cavity. You can have this test done as an outpatient without an anaesthetic; any discomfort is short lived. Only a tiny piece of material is needed to send to the laboratory, where it is examined for any secretory changes.

Unfortunately, as with virtually all ways of checking ovulation, EB is not a foolproof way of detecting ovulation. You may produce enough progesterone to cause secretory changes even without ovulating. Alternatively, a few women have a damaged endometrium which just does not become secretory even though ovulation has taken place.

Laparoscopy

The laparoscope may be used during the second half of the cycle, some time after you are thought to have ovulated. This is a telescope several inches long and about as thick as a fountain pen, which is inserted into the abdomen. You are given a general anaesthetic and the telescope is introduced through a tiny hole made in your navel. This leaves a minute scar, which is almost invisible. A powerful light is shone down the telescope and the surgeon can get an accurate view of the tubes, the outside of the uterus and the ovaries. Other organs, such as your appendix and liver, can be examined at the same time.

The ovaries can be seen clearly with this telescope and it is usually quite obvious when an ovary has ovulated. The follicle the egg was shed from contains large blood vessels and is a yellowish colour. The yellow follicle is called a corpus luteum (Latin, meaning yellow body) and a small hole will probably be seen in it. This is the point where the egg escaped and so it is good evidence of ovulation. But because it requires a general anaesthetic this is another test used mostly when others haven't provided results.

Most women feel bloated and a little uncomfortable for twenty-four hours after a laparoscopy. You may also have discomfort in the chest and some pain around the shoulder due to the gas which is injected into the abdomen. This tends to irritate the nerves supplying the abdomen and chest wall. But the discomfort does not last long and most people find they can perform normal activities within twenty-four to forty-eight hours afterwards. The main problem is usually a rather sore throat, which is caused by the tube that the anaesthetist uses to give a really safe anaesthetic.

What are the risks of laparoscopy? These are minimal in good hands. A tiny proportion of women have some internal bleeding (about two per thousand). This hardly ever requires further treatment. An equally tiny proportion of people may suffer bowel perforation when the telescopic equipment is introduced, and very rarely an immediate operation will be needed to repair the damage. It must be emphasized that this is truly exceptional – in the last five thousand laparoscopies done in our unit this has been necessary just once. This woman came to no harm, and conceived five months later without complications.

Could an endometrial biopsy or laparoscopy affect an early pregnancy? Naturally there is always the worry that if you have a test such as laparoscopy or endometrial biopsy in the second half of your cycle, the doctor might damage an early pregnancy. It is rather unlikely that a laparoscopy will damage an early pregnancy, and I can remember this only once in the many thousands of laparoscopies that I have done. This woman miscarried, but fortunately had another pregnancy shortly afterwards.

The risks of endometrial biopsy are also slight, and I know of several women who had perfectly normal pregnancies after biopsies during the first few weeks when they were pregnant. There seems to be no risk of having an abnormal baby – if there is any at all, it is confined to miscarriage. We are convinced that the benefits of these tests greatly outweigh the risks.

Ovarian biopsy

Very occasionally during laparoscopy, if there is a suspicion that a woman's ovary has no eggs in it, the doctor may take a small piece of the outer skin of the ovary. This can be studied later and any undeveloped follicles containing eggs in them counted. This test is useful in the rare conditions when very few or no eggs at all are produced, when the diagnosis of complete ovarian failure may be reached.

TREATMENT

For most problems with ovulation, the treatment is now astonishingly effective. It should be very easy to stimulate your ovaries if you are not ovulating; in fact, there is a better than 90 per cent chance that your ovaries can be made to work properly with the right drug. You may wonder whether the risks of multiple birth will be a problem if taking drugs is suggested for you. Although this still occasionally happens, nowadays we are far more able to control the way the drugs work.

For the few women with complete ovarian failure, it is unlikely we can start eggs being produced again, so the outlook is not good. This is a disappointment that has to be faced, and I discuss ways of dealing with it in Chapters 11 and 12.

Treating failure of ovulation with drugs

The most commonly used drug is clomiphene (usually known as Clomid or Serophene). The history of its discovery may interest you. During research for new contraceptives many years ago, it was realized that estrogen (in the form of the contraceptive pill) prevented ovulation. However, estrogen tended to cause complications, so some drug companies began to search for a pill that acted like estrogen on the body but without side effects. One chemical they looked at was clomiphene. Although clomiphene was free of side effects, hopes for it as a substitute for estrogen were dashed when researchers found that rats given it bred perfectly normally. The drug was put on the shelf for years because no one could think of any use for it. Then researchers looking at earlier records noted that those very rats had actually got pregnant remarkably readily. Someone had a bright idea – maybe clomiphene could be used to increase fertility. Luckily for many thousands of women, this unusual compound was found to promote ovulation.

Clomiphene is now used on a massive scale. It has had such a success that it has sometimes been given when it really isn't necessary. You should not take clomiphene unless you have proof you are not ovulating, because some normally ovulating women become temporarily infertile with it. It should always be given by a doctor, with regular checks to confirm that eggs are in fact leaving the ovary. The usual dosage is one pill every day for five days near the beginning of the menstrual cycle, about two to five days after your period starts.

Clomiphene seems to get the pituitary gland to work harder, so stimulating the ovary. Sometimes it can affect the cervical mucus, making it difficult for the sperm to penetrate it. Clomiphene may also interfere with the development of the uterus lining (the endometrium – see page 11). This is the main reason why it is given early in the cycle, so that your mucus and uterus have time to recover before ovulation and possible conception. Side effects with clomiphene are very uncommon. A few women may bleed irregularly. You may feel a little unwell, and very occasionally a few women get hot flushes when taking these pills. Since you are taking them for a limited time, these effects are hardly worth bothering about.

Other drugs that are similar to clomiphene There are several other pills that you may be prescribed if clomiphene does not work in your case. The commonest are tamoxifen and cyclofenil. These are very like clomiphene in action, and are taken in a similar way. They have few special advantages and are only occasionally more effective than clomiphene. They work in about 5 to 10 per cent of women who don't respond to clomiphene.

Human chorionic gonadotrophin (HCG) This is a substance similar to LH, the main hormone that is produced at the time of ovulation by the pituitary gland (see page 9). HCG is given to you as an injection, usually in combination with clomiphene, just before ovulation is expected. It is not much help by itself, but together with clomiphene it encourages the ovary to burst the follicle which contains the egg. You should have HCG prescribed only if it has been found that you have this problem of the egg not escaping from the follicle. HCG should be taken at exactly the right time in your cycle, under close supervision from your doctor. If it is given too early in the cycle it may actually interfere with ovulation, preventing conception both that month and the next. For this reason it has to be injected in the middle of the cycle, on or around the fourteenth day after your period begins.

Human menopausal gonadotrophin (HMG) This is the so-called fertility drug, and is very powerful (it is known by one of its trade names, Humegon or Pergonal). It contains a mixture of the pituitary hormones LH and FSH in about equal quantities. The way it is manufactured may surprise you. Women produce large amounts of LH and FSH every day at the time of the menopause, because the ovaries are starting to fail. The pituitary gland detects this failure because the amount of estrogen produced by the ovaries falls. The pituitary compensates by pouring out more and more FSH and LH in an attempt to get the ovary to work better. This excess of pituitary hormone is not used and passes out of the body via the urine. Pergonal is made from the pooled urine taken from nunneries where there are large numbers of menopausal women. It is then purified and packaged. This is quite a complex chemical process, and HMG is an expensive drug.

You may be offered Pergonal or Humegon if clomiphene treatment has been unsuccessful. Injections are usually given repeatedly for several days during the first half of the cycle. It encourages the ovaries to produce several follicles containing eggs, and so there is a risk of a lot of eggs being produced in the same cycle; this is why some women have twins or even more conceptions with it. So Pergonal has to be given under the closest supervision. Regular hormone tests on your blood or urine are needed during treatment, as people have different responses. With the correct supervision it is possible to make sure that just enough follicles are being stimulated. Ultrasound is often used to check what is happening, and this way of detecting multiple ovulation normally prevents any serious risk of more than one baby.

The main advantage of HMG is that it is very effective, and unless your ovaries have failed completely, it is usually possible to stimulate ovulation once the correct dose has been decided.

Pure follicle stimulating hormone (FSH) A highly effective alternative to HMG has recently been developed. Pergonal and Humegon contain both FSH and LH, but actually it is the FSH that is the active part of this drug. The LH is not always needed in such high concentrations and LH given at the same time as FSH may interfere with ovarian function in certain women. The problem has been that until very recently it wasn't possible to manufacture pure FSH.

Purified FSH is given by injection like HMG and needs careful supervision. It is sometimes more useful for women with polycystic ovarian disease or Stein-Leventhal syndrome (see p. 50), if Pergonal has not been effective.

Recombinant FSH FSH is now being made by genetic engineering. Currently, genetically engineered FSH is only available on a restricted basis, but it has the substantial advantage that it is a very pure form of FSH. This makes it safer to use, and it is very likely that trials will show that the improved effectiveness of this drug justifies its extra expense. At the time of writing, this drug has not been costed, but it is likely to be rather more expensive than other FSH preparations.

The side effects of FSH treatments All these drugs vigorously stimulate the ovaries. Occasionally (in about one in a hundred cases) they can lead to the ovaries being overstimulated. This is why careful monitoring with ultrasound should always be employed when they are being used. Hyperstimulation can lead to pain in the ovaries, and occasionally swelling of the tummy due to accumulation of fluid in the abdomen. This can be sufficiently serious to justify bed rest in hospital in a few cases. Many women have been made very anxious about rumours suggesting that FSH treatments might cause ovarian cancers; there is absolutely no real evidence that this is a genuine risk, and extensive experience with the class of drugs over more than thirty years lead nearly all experts to believe that people have been unnecessarily scared by these stories.

Releasing hormones and pump therapy (GnRH)   Another recent development is treatment with repeated injections of gonado-trophin releasing hormones (GnRH). These are the hormones made by the hypothalamus (see page 9) that cause the release of LH and FSH from the pituitary gland. Now that these hormones can be manufactured they can be given in certain cases instead of HMG or FSH.

The hypothalamus secretes releasing hormones in a pulsatile fashion – that is, it secretes small amounts intermittently every fifteen minutes or so. The frequency of these pulses is important and if GnRH is given as a drug, it also needs to be given in frequent regular pulses to mimic the hypothalamus and thus 'fool' the pituitary gland into producing LH and FSH in a natural manner. Obviously, to give a person an injection every fifteen minutes would be unpleasant to say the least, so to get over this problem, the pump was developed. This is a small device about the size of a cigarette carton which can be attached to the upper arm, with a tiny tube going into a small vein. The pump can be worn night and day without discomfort – indeed, after a while people forget it is there – and it can give intermittent doses of GnRH for several days, if needed. This treatment is often effective if you have polycystic ovaries not responding to conventional treatment. It has the advantage that the side effects of HMG or FSH treatment are less likely. Moreover, it usually stimulates only one follicle in the ovary, and the risk of twins is therefore much less.

Bromocriptine   This works quite differently as, strictly speaking, it does not stimulate ovulation by itself. It prevents the pituitary gland from making too much prolactin, the milk producing hormone. So you will be given bromocriptine only if you are producing excess prolactin. You may need to take these tablets for several months at a time, and your doctor will probably check that it is producing the desired effect by measuring your prolactin in blood samples before and during treatment. You may feel a little faint or giddy in the first week or two, but these feelings rapidly disappear. Because of the possibility of these early side effects you should avoid driving a car for a few days after starting the drug, until you are certain that you are no longer having any trouble.

Progesterone You may have a problem at ovulation time even though you menstruate regularly and shed an egg from your ovaries. This may be because you are not making enough progesterone after ovulation has occurred, so that the embryo fails to implant (see also page 11). Injections of pure progesterone after ovulation may help. Some doctors prefer to prescribe the progesterone in the form of a vaginal pessary, which seems to be equally effective. This treatment is not very widespread, as there is some doubt about whether it really is effective.

Corticosteroids It has been well known for years that some infertile women conceive immediately after being given corticosteroids – the drugs that are prescribed for inflammatory problems (including arthritis and acne). Steroids are now a rare treatment for infertility, and have been almost completely replaced by the various drugs I've already described. Why they should stimulate the ovaries is not entirely clear. Corticosteroid treatment may still help, however, if it is discovered that you are not ovulating because you are producing too much male hormone. It is not always realized that all normal women produce male hormone (testosterone) as well as female hormone. Your adrenal gland (situated above your kidneys) may produce too much of it, in which case corticosteroids may be prescribed to reduce the amount you make.

Other hormonal treatments Various other hormone treatments have been tried in the past. Few, if any, have stood the test of time. The only ones still given are thyroid hormone pills, and generally with very little scientific basis. They are really effective only for women with a thyroid disorder, which is a rare cause of infertility. For normal women to take thyroid as a treatment may actually be dangerous, and it should not be given without strong evidence that you have decreased thyroid function.

How long will you need to continue treatment?

Each drug is different and one woman's response isn't always the same as another's; you may have to try several drugs. It usually takes several months for any one treatment to succeed.

If your doctor is sure that you are ovulating only when you are taking drugs, you should keep trying – unless the treatment is very distressing to you. Some women do not get pregnant for very many months after starting clomiphene or Pergonal, even though tests confirm that they are ovulating. I know of many patients who had ovulation stimulated for two or even three years before they finally became pregnant. As far as I know, the world record for Pergonal is thirty-eight months of treatment, followed by a normal pregnancy; and I have seen several women who took clomiphene for even longer, eventually with success. If you are having trouble, it might be worth trying to take these drugs every alternate month as some women finally conceive in the months in between treatment.

Operations for polycystic ovaries

In exceptional circumstances, particularly if the ovaries tend to form small cysts and drugs will not force them to ovulate, some doctors recommend an operation on the ovaries themselves.

Polycystic ovarian disease is an odd problem, which can cause infertility. In 1933, two gynaecologists, Dr Irvine Stein and Dr Michael Leventhal, noted that some women who did not ovulate and who had no periods had ovaries that were rather enlarged and contained cysts. Some were also overweight and had excessive hair, especially on their face and chest. This condition, which is really of unknown cause, came to be called the Stein-Leventhal syndrome, after the two doctors who first described it in detail. They suggested removing a piece of each ovary to confirm the diagnosis of cysts. Purely by chance, it was found that when pieces of the ovaries were removed, some of the women started to ovulate. This discovery led to treatment by ovarian 'wedge resection', in which a small slice is taken from each ovary and the sliced area is then stitched back together. This operation was done much more often in the days before effective drug treatment had been discovered. It can be surprisingly effective, but nowadays it will be suggested for you only if all treatment with tablets of clomiphene and injections such as pure FSH has failed and yet your ovaries still have a chance of working. Why it should work at all is something of a mystery, but the reason may be that removal of a small segment of ovarian tissue helps prevent overproduction of hormones and so reestablishes normal ovulation.

The operation is considered a minor one, and you are unlikely to have any serious after effects. You will have a scar about 6 in (15 cm) long in the lower part of your abdomen, which will be quite unnoticeable after a few months. You will be able to have intercourse again within three weeks.

A recently developed alternative to wedge resection of the ovaries, is laparoscopic ovarian diathermy. In this procedure, the surgeon punctures the little cystic follicles in the ovaries using an electrical needle or a laser. It has the very great advantage that it avoids an open operation and it is possible to leave hospital the following day after surgery, with much less discomfort. At the time of writing, it is unclear just how successful this procedure really is, but certainly we have seen a number of women whose ovaries have ovulated spontaneously for up to nine months after this quick operation. It may also make any drug treatment more effective.

After all these tests and attempts with treatment you may finally be told you have complete ovarian failure. Is there no hope? It is true that there is no known treatment (apart possibly from egg donation, see Chapter 11) if your ovaries have failed and have no eggs in them. However, ovarian failure is a very curious disorder, and it does seem that sometimes the ovaries just 'go to sleep'. There are rare examples of a very few women returning to absolutely normal ovarian function years after failure has been diagnosed, starting to menstruate normally and shedding eggs. The diagnosis of ovarian failure does not absolutely mean that you will be sterile for ever. Unfortunately, there is no treatment that can speed things up and it seems to be a question of luck whether this will happen. You have to face this with a lot of patience and try not to hold on to false hopes.

How do you know if you have started to ovulate spontaneously? You can only guess, if you detect the signs described on page 34. If in doubt, it may be worth asking your doctor for tests. But I hardly need say, you do not have to wait before trying for a baby.

4

Tubal disease and endometriosis

In this chapter I describe two very common conditions and their treatment. The first, tubal damage, has a direct bearing on fertility, while the connection between endometriosis and infertility is less certain.

TUBAL DISEASE

Although having blocked tubes is often believed by women to be the reason for their trouble, it is not the commonest cause of infertility. Tubal disease involves problems other than blockage, and all these together amount to approximately one third of female infertility.

Unfortunately and quite wrongly, some doctors regard tubal damage as hopeless, and they may dissuade women from seeking the best advice. Even the most complicated problems can be treated, so do not be discouraged. This is probably the most specialized branch of infertility treatment. The results tend not to be good except in skilled hands; if it is suggested for you, it is sensible to insist on going to a major centre where there is a large volume of this kind of work so that you get a really reliable opinion and the best treatment.

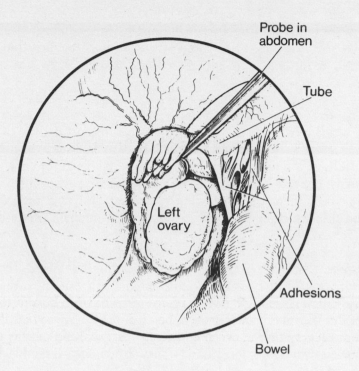

Adhesions, seen here between the left tube and bowel

You need not worry that a tubal problem will damage your health if it is not treated. Tubal disease is very benign and seldom, if ever, threatens general health. The only reason you may consider the tubal surgery described in this chapter is if you want to maximize your chances of having a baby. Tubal damage that may cause infertility includes:

Complete blockage of the tubes at one or more points. Generally, tubal blockage affects both tubes equally and symmetrically. This means that if one tube is blocked, the other will be too, and usually at the same spot. Women are often diagnosed during first tests as having completely blocked tubes, of course implying that they are infertile. However, this diagnosis may later on be found to be incorrect; total blockage is the least common type of tubal damage.

Narrowing or partial blockage of the tubes because of scarring. This is seen mostly after infection. Again, this kind of damage usually affects both tubes equally, but it may be possible to conceive, as an egg may slip past the narrowed area into the uterus.

Damage to the lining of the tubes or the muscle wall usually as a result of an infection. This is much more common than is often thought, and can happen whether the tubes are blocked or not. The lining cells of the tube, which have microscopic hairs, or cilia, are extremely delicate and easily damaged. Scarring after infection may prevent them from working properly. This is a little like scarred skin which may stop sweating or growing hair after a bad burn.

Adhesions that have formed usually around the tubes. Tissue grows in an area that has been damaged and can glue the tubes to nearby structures, such as the ovaries, uterus or bowel. Adhesions may splint the tubes and stop them being able to move so that they may not pick up an egg or carry it to the uterus. People often ask what these adhesions look like – they frequently resemble the strands of glue you can see between pieces of paper that have been pulled slightly apart when the glue was not yet hard.

WHAT CAUSES TUBAL DAMAGE?

Inflammation

It seems that the number of people who suffer with tubal disease is increasing; this, if true, is probably for several reasons. Most, but not all, tubal problems are due to an earlier infection (called pelvic inflammatory disease, which may follow salpingitis – infection of the tubes). This may be caused by a wide range of bacteria, most of them common germs we all carry in our bodies, which usually cause no problems at all. For reasons that are still not clearly understood, these bacteria multiply rapidly in some women to cause scarring and sometimes blockage.

People are wrongly inclined to think that tubal disease is always caused by venereal (or sexually transmitted) infection. Venereal disease is only one cause of tubal damage and not the most usual. It is true, though, that it is very unusual for virgins to have tubal infection. Infection is also uncommon among women who have had sex with only one partner. So sexual activity does play an important part in the development of some cases of pelvic inflammatory disease.

You may wonder how you caught an infection and particularly whether your partner was responsible. 'Did I get my tubal infection from my partner?' is a question many women want to ask – but leave unspoken. The answer is almost certainly no. In our clinic, where a wide range of tubal problems are seen, only about 5 per cent of infections can be traced back to sexual contact. As I have said, it is true that sexual activity, in general, makes women more prone to pelvic infection. It is also true that walking about on a cold night without an overcoat makes some people prone to influenza.

Factors that may lead to scarring of the tubes also include:

The coil or intrauterine contraceptive device (IUD)

Wearing a coil sometimes leads to infection in the uterine cavity, which can spread to the tubes. Women who have symptoms such as irregular bleeding or bad pelvic pain when wearing a coil seem more likely to get pelvic inflammation. It is our impression that infection is also more likely among women who wear a coil who have never been pregnant. For this reason, we advise women who have not had a child to avoid this method of contraception.

Infection in the abdominal cavity

There are a number of infections that start in the abdomen and can spread to the fallopian tubes. For example, very occasionally women have tubal damage after appendicitis or other illnesses involving the intestine.

Inflammation after the delivery of a baby

Many women who suffer with secondary infertility – that is, infertility after having had one baby – have had some form of infection in the first few weeks after delivery, when their uterus and tubes are most susceptible to inflammation. Although this is not the most common cause, a substantial number of women do have this problem; an estimated 15 per cent of tubal infections may be due to it.

Inflammation after miscarriage or abortion

This is a frequent cause of tubal damage, and is similar to inflammation after having a baby. Before abortion was legalized, backstreet abortion was much more common. This kind of infection was more frequent then and often more serious in its consequences. Around 10 to 15 per cent of infections may still be the result of miscarriage or abortion.

If you were unfortunate enough to have had an abortion you may worry, probably wrongly, that you have brought infertility on yourself. In any case, this event is firmly in the past. It really does not help to feel guilt or self-recrimination about something that almost certainly happened several years earlier and about events that, at the time, you had little ability to control. People very understandably often feel guilty about the past; very often these natural feelings distort what really happened. It is important to keep your feelings in perspective. You'll probably find it is best for you and your partner to draw a line under the past and look positively on what now can be done.

Surgery

An operation involving the uterus and tubes can cause adhesions to form (see above). Very rarely this follows the curettage operation D and C, see page 87).

Previous ectopic pregnancy (see Chapter 7)

When a fertilized egg implants itself in the fallopian tubes, it may begin to grow, so becoming an ectopic pregnancy (outside the uterus). The place in the tube where the implantation happened becomes scarred and an area of calcification – like a little stone in the tube – may form. The first a woman may know of an ectopic pregnancy that happened many years earlier is subsequent tests showing that one tube is blocked. Normally, though, ectopic pregnancy is diagnosed and treated immediately it occurs. Nearly always blockage from an ectopic pregnancy is on one side only.

Congenital abnormalities

A very few women have abnormal development of their tubes from before birth and are born with one or both blocked or absent. The uterus may also be abnormal in these cases (see page 84).

Endometriosis

This can lead to scarring of the tubes, adhesions and, in severe cases, to tubal blockage. (See page 74.)

HOW CAN I TELL IF MY TUBES ARE DAMAGED?

It is unlikely that you will know until this has been investigated by your doctor. Tubal infection often causes very few symptoms, so most women are unaware of the problem until they try for a baby. Few have any clear idea that they have had tubal infection in the past but there are some clues:

- Some women remember an episode of acute pelvic pain and tenderness, which may have been accompanied by vaginal discharge and a high temperature. This may mean they had an attack of salpingitis. Usually an infection of this sort is cleared, with or without antibiotics, and there are no further problems. A few women turn out to be infertile, often years later. They have had salpingitis that has resulted in scarring and adhesions involving the tubes.
- Some other women remember that they had a fairly long period of pain and irregular bleeding after having a baby or mis-carriage.
- A few who have had venereal disease, usually gonorrhoea, may be affected. But as already emphasized, it is important to

realize that most women who have had venereal disease remain fertile.

- Endometriosis or chronic inflammation may cause quite severe pain or tenderness during intercourse. Curiously, the severity of symptoms does not always relate to the degree of damage. Women with no symptoms may have extensive endometriosis, while others with bad discomfort may have only mild disease.
- Dysmenorrhoea – bad period pain – is another symptom of both endometriosis and inflammation. Of course, period pains are very common and the majority of women with dysmenorrhoea are completely healthy. Sometimes, endometriosis may cause pain on passing urine or opening the bowels. Again, the amount of discomfort bears little relationship to the likelihood of infertility, and women with crippling pain may conceive without difficulty.

Congenital problems do not often produce symptoms you can detect. Just occasionally a problem in the uterus will cause painful or abnormal periods. Otherwise a congenital abnormality will be discovered only when tests are done. Your doctor will send you to the hospital for tests if tubal damage seems likely.

Tests to detect tubal damage

Although a few women feel tenderness in their pelvis when they have a full internal examination by their doctor, tubal disease cannot usually be discovered during a routine examination. Tests will have to be done in hospital.

Insufflation   Some doctors used to blow gas through the tubes to see if they are open. This was really rather unreliable, and often painful. It had the advantage of being very quick and easy as the gas is blown in from below by a small pipe inserted into the cervix. However, many women found it a distressing procedure. Because of this and because a negative test does not necessarily mean your tubes really are blocked, we have now completely abandoned it in our own clinic.

X-rays   An x-ray of the uterus and tubes can be taken, normally as an outpatient. This is called a hysterosalpingogram (often referred to as HSG for short). It is very useful as it gives information not gained by other tests. A teaspoonful of special dye is injected into the uterus from below and is allowed to trickle into the tubes. This dye looks like water but is opaque to x-rays and shows up on an x-ray screen as a white area. If your tubes are blocked or constricted, the dye will not enter them, and an obvious deformity will be seen on the x-ray photograph. Although many doctors rely on laparoscopy (see below) because this gives a direct view of the tubes, x-rays are invaluable and cannot be replaced. Deformities *inside* the tube can be seen only on an x-ray; besides, x-rays show the state of your uterine cavity, which is not easily assessed by other methods.

Unpleasant and inaccurate stories about tubal x-rays frighten women quite needlessly. Most think that a hysterosalpingogram will cause pain. Although this is better done without an anaesthetic as we nearly always get more information and better pictures, there shouldn't be any pain provided the procedure is done gently and the dye is injected really slowly. About 25 per cent of women who have an x-ray have a little momentary discomfort, but this passes off after ten minutes or so; it should never be unbearable.

What are the risks of hysterosalpingography? The main risk is of starting up old infections, but this is very slight indeed providing sensible precautions are taken. A hysterosalpingogram should be postponed if:

- you feel a lot of tenderness when you have a pelvic examination
- you have had some recently increasing pain on sexual intercourse
- you have a bad vaginal discharge
- you have suffered a bad attack of salpingitis within the three preceding months
- your doctor considers you are at high risk of further inflammation. You should be given antibiotics for a few days before x-ray
- you are menstruating, when your uterus is more susceptible to infection.

Laparoscopy (see also Chapter 3) is important for detecting tubal disease, because no other test gives a really good view of adhesions or damage to the outside of the tubes. It is always done if we suspect endometriosis (see later). During laparoscopy coloured dye is injected into your tubes to show up any blockage. However, it cannot replace x-rays, and if tubal disease is confirmed, you will almost certainly need both tests. Laparoscopy should be done by someone skilled in infertility surgery to ensure the maximum information is gained. It has a unique advantage as it can be used as a treatment as well as a test. Adhesions can sometimes be divided just using the telescope, avoiding further surgery. Some surgeons even use the laparoscope to open blocked tubes, employing a laser or very fine laparoscopic scissors to operate on the ends of the tubes. However laparoscopic surgery does not seem to give as good results as open surgery using a microscope.

If something more fundamental needs to be done and an open operation is indicated, you may want to have it all completed under the same anaesthetic. However, although it is possible to perform tubal surgery immediately if a blockage is found, it is generally not the best thing to do. Even if it does seem inconvenient to have a second anaesthetic, there are several good reasons for not having tubal surgery immediately after laparoscopy:

- Tubal operations are quite complicated and really need careful planning for the best chance of pregnancy. It is usually easier to schedule them properly in advance when a laparoscopy has already been done.
- Laparoscopy tends to irritate the tissues slightly and if surgery is done immediately healing may take longer. A gap of at least one week between the two procedures is best.
- Good surgeons like to have the opportunity of a proper discussion with the couple about tubal surgery. It usually pays handsomely if you are able to ask exactly what was found during your laparoscopy before you agree to an operation. Better knowledge of your situation will help you appreciate the advantages and disadvantages of future surgery.

TREATMENT FOR TUBAL DISEASE

Treatment with drugs

Except in one or two very special circumstances, there are at present no satisfactory drug treatments for tubal damage. Drug treatments occasionally work if the tubes are blocked because of endometriosis (see below).

Tubal washouts (or hydrotubation)

Blocked fallopian tubes have been treated by fluid or gas being injected forcibly through them from below. This is risky and not often done nowadays because there is a real chance of bacteria being spread from the vagina. This treatment is also often painful, and there is not much evidence of its success. We do not use it in our clinic.

Tubal surgery – for which conditions would you need it?

The investigations described above will have shown where and how badly your tubes are affected. Surgery may be suggested if you have any of these problems:

1. Adhesions around the tubes. This is possibly the commonest problem, and an operation can be done to remove the adhesions. The technical name for this is adhesiolysis or salpingolysis (from the Greek *salpingos*, meaning tube and *lysis*, Greek for freeing). If there is little damage to the tubes themselves, the success rate is around 45 per cent. When adhesions are severe and the tubes not badly damaged, it is about 35 to 40 per cent. The chances of pregnancy tend to be better when the adhesions are due to endometriosis than when due to inflammation.

2. Complete blockage of the outer end of the tube. Infection may lead to total blockage of the tube at its outer end, near the ovary (see the diagram on page 14). The operation to open tubes damaged in this way is called salpingostomy (*stoma* means

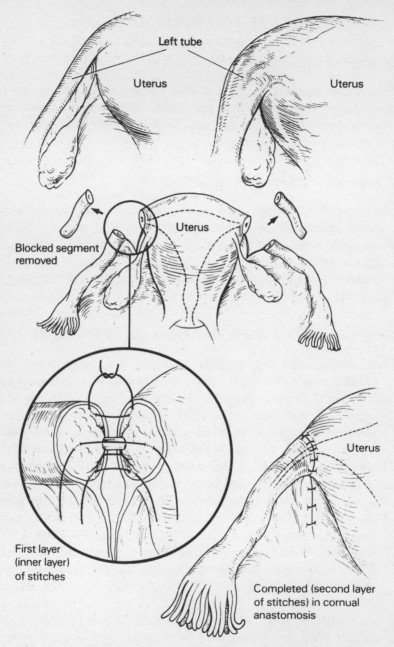

A blockage where the tube joins the uterus at the cornu, causing an enlargement of the area, and cornual anastomosis to remove this

mouth or opening). Salpingostomy done with microsurgery (the operation is performed with the use of a microscope, see page 64) will result in permanent unblocking of the tubes in about 90 per cent of cases. However, far fewer women than this actually get pregnant because the blockage is usually associated with severe damage to the lining of the tube and the muscle wall, which often do not heal even after the tubes have been unblocked. Among women with damage that is not bad, up to 30 to 40 per cent may conceive. However, in most cases it is severe, so the overall success rate is about 18 to 25 per cent.

3. Incomplete blockage of the outer end of the tube. The tube may be scarred and narrowed at its outer end without being completely blocked. Operations to reconstruct the unblocked end of the tube will reshape the fimbria (*fimbria* is Latin for edge or fringe). The operation is called fimbrioplasty. Often the damage to the tube itself is less severe than when the tube is completely blocked and the surgical results are better. About 40 to 45 per cent of these operations may result in a successful pregnancy.

4. Blockage where the tube joins the uterus, at its narrowest part (see the diagram on page 62). This may happen after infection with a coil or following pregnancy or miscarriage. If the part of the tube is undamaged in the wall of the uterus, it is possible to cut out the blocked section and rejoin the tube. This operation, which is technically very difficult, is called cornual anastomosis (the cornua being the corners of the uterus – *cornu* is Latin for a horn and *anastomosis* means a join). When done by microsurgery (see below) up to 60 per cent of women become pregnant afterwards. Occasionally the block may be so extensive that the damage extends right through the wall of the uterus into the uterine cavity. If this is the situation, the tube can be implanted through a new hole bored into the uterus. This operation, called tubal implantation, used to be done more frequently when cornual anastomosis was still experimental. It carries about a 25 per cent chance of success, and nowadays should be used only when the damage cannot be treated by the more specialized technique of anastomosis.

5. Endometriosis which is suspected of causing a blockage or extensive scarring (see later).

6. Reversal of sterilization (see Chapter 8).

What have you got to lose by having surgery?　Although surgery is the most successful treatment for blocked tubes, you should think carefully before going in for it. If you have tubal disease, no matter how good your treatment, you are unlikely to have even as much as a 50 per cent chance of having a child of your own. If your tubes are blocked and you decide against surgery, you can be virtually certain that you will not get pregnant; it may be possible to come to terms with this. If you have an operation on your tubes, you don't know whether you will become pregnant or not. Therefore each menstrual period after the operation can become a very stressful time. It is even worse if, for some reason, your period is delayed for a few days.

I shall never forget one delightful (and very stable) woman who told me about two years after I had operated on her tubes, 'I wa fine before my operation – I knew I could not get pregnant ana learned to live with it. Once you had operated on me, I didn't know where I stood any more and I became very depressed. I've come to terms with this now, but I've had two miserably difficult years.'

Will the tubal problem get worse if it is not treated immediately? This depends on the kind of tubal damage you have. If the outer end of the tube is blocked completely and you have a hydrosalpinx (water on the tube), the accumulated fluid may not escape. The build-up of this fluid will cause gradual deterioration of the tubal wall and lining over several years. Therefore, if this is your situation, it is better to have surgery sooner rather than later. All other forms of tubal disease do not seem to be progressive in this way, and as we have already said, they will not damage your health in other ways, so there is no urgency.

The operations

The results of tubal surgery have continued to improve recently, largely because of the introduction of microsurgery – surgery done

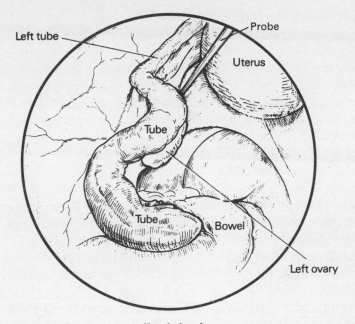

Hydrosalpinx, showing a swollen left tube

with the aid of a special microscope. The microscope is invaluable because of the tiny dimensions of the human fallopian tubes. The internal diameter at its narrowest part is only 0.5 millimetre – about the thickness of a piece of button thread. The microscope is of enormous help if a pipe this thin is to be stitched together accurately; also because it helps the surgeon avoid damage to surrounding delicate structures. This reduces the risk of adhesions, which used to be the main cause of failure of these operations. Tubal surgery, though, does require an incision in the abdominal wall. Tubal microsurgery must be considered major surgery, and you have to stay in hospital for three to seven days afterwards.

Recently there has been great publicity about lasers being used for tubal microsurgery. The advantages claimed for them include better healing after surgery and even less risk of adhesion formation. At present there seems to be little evidence for these claims and the general impression among infertility surgeons is that the laser offers few, if any, advantages. You certainly do not stand an increased chance of having a baby after laser surgery.

Tubal surgery done down the laparoscope

Although not all cases of tubal disease are suitable for this method of surgery it is increasingly clear that many women may benefit from this approach – particularly when their tubes are not totally blocked. The major advantage is that the stay in hospital is much shorter, one or two days only. Another advantage is that a bigger incision in the abdominal wall is avoided and pain and discomfort are reduced. Recovery is also more rapid. However, there is no evidence at all yet that the chances of pregnancy are better, or even as good.

What are the risks of tubal surgery? The physical risks are small. There are extremely few complications and the overall risk of damage to your health is less than one in five hundred, because women having tubal surgery are generally very fit physically. It is statistically safer than any other form of gynaecological surgery, and complications such as a chest infection, blood clots in the leg veins and abdominal problems are very uncommon. There are, though, a few longer term difficulties to be noted:

- Any woman with damaged tubes has an increased risk of an ectopic pregnancy (see page 114). This is greater after tubal surgery, because by opening the tubes the surgeon increases the chance of all types of conception.
- There is a very slight risk of increased pelvic pain after surgery. Some women suffer from pelvic pain before tubal surgery. This can be due to adhesion formation around the ovaries, although the precise reason is not often clear. For most women, tubal surgery much more frequently reduces pain associated with tubal disease.
- As I have explained, there is a substantial chance that the surgery will not result in a successful pregnancy and you therefore risk disappointment.

When it comes to having surgery, you may think you'd be better off with the test-tube baby technique – that your chances of success are higher. I would always recommend tubal surgery where both alternatives are available and the tubes are not badly damaged, for the following reasons:

- Conception can occur naturally in a normal menstrual cycle, when you are not particularly expecting it, and after natural sexual intercourse.
- Tubal surgery offers a chance of permanent restoration of fertility without further treatment. Many women coming to our clinic have now had a second or third or even fourth normal pregnancy without needing to consult a doctor again.
- Most women seem to find that tubal surgery is easier to bear. A major problem with in vitro fertilization is the stress that is involved during each treatment cycle.
- Tubal surgery often has much better success rates, particularly in skilled hands and especially if the patient has not already had major pelvic operations.
- The chances of a miscarriage may be lower.

I describe in vitro fertilization in more detail in Chapter 10. Sometimes people ask me if there are any newer types of surgery that can be tried:

Can you replace my tubes with a plastic pipe? The fallopian tube is one of the most complex tubular structures in the human body. It is not simply a drainpipe for the egg to roll down into the uterus. Among its delicate functions are:

- Capture of the egg from the ovary.
- Transport of the egg to the site of fertilization, in the middle section of the tube.
- Transport of the sperm up the tube towards the site of fertilization. Amazingly, the tube transports the sperm in one direction while transporting the egg in the other *at the same time*.
- It provides the precise amount of chemicals needed for fertilization and early embryo growth.
- The tube removes waste products from the developing embryo.
- It protects the embryo for the first three days of life and times its move into the uterus so exactly that it arrives at the best stage of development for later implantation.

Clearly the tube could not effectively be replaced by a piece of plastic or indeed by other living tissue.

Could I have a tubal transplant?   Because of the complex nature of the tube and the fact that it is sometimes hopelessly damaged, some scientists and physicians have experimented with transplantation of a tube from a healthy donor. There have been no successes. It is technically a very difficult operation and there is usually a need to take potentially dangerous drugs afterwards to prevent the tube being rejected. Test-tube baby treatment is likely to be a much better bet.

Other worries that you may have are:

Your age   It becomes increasingly difficult to justify tubal surgery after the age of about forty. There are few successes after that because fertility is so reduced by then. The oldest successful patient I know is a woman who had surgery at forty-four and conceived five months later. Her case sticks in the mind because her story is unusual.

Your cycle   Is there any time during the menstrual cycle when tubal surgery should not be done? No. There are many myths about this, but no real information that it makes any difference. It is usually best not to operate while you are actually menstruating, simply because surgery is marginally easier at other times. There is a theoretical risk of endometriosis if certain types of surgery are done during a period, but this is very slight.

The scar   Tubal surgery is usually done through a cut across the lower abdomen, that is, in the hairline below the suntan mark made by a brief bikini. This means that the scar will not be visible except to your nearest and dearest. Because these incisions nearly always heal so well, the scar will probably not be very obvious even when you are completely undressed.

Drugs you may need

Antibiotics   Because recurrent infection is a serious cause of failure of tubal surgery, most doctors like to give antibiotics for the first few days after the operation. We normally start these drugs on the day of the operation, and continue to give the tablets for three to seven days.

Steroids These cortisone-like drugs may be given immediately after surgery for up to one week. They sometimes help to reduce adhesion formation because they slow down the healing process. They may produce a little temporary weight gain as they cause your body to retain fluid, but the main problem is that wound healing may also be slightly delayed. Serious side effects are rare and the fluid is lost once the steroids are stopped.

Anti-inflammatory drugs These, too, are to reduce adhesion formation. They may have a side effect of being like a sedative, so that they reduce discomfort but make you a little sleepy. These drugs are more widely used in North America than in Britain.

Painkillers These are usually needed only for the first forty-eight hours after the operation. After that serious discomfort is very uncommon, although most women suffer with wind for a few days.

After the operation

Although you are likely to feel far better than you expected immediately after surgery, all abdominal operations need a period of convalescence. There is usually very little discomfort, but most people find that they feel more tired than they had expected. A few women return to work within three weeks of surgery, but this is not common. Most need a month, and a few six weeks.

Heavy lifting and very vigorous exercise should be avoided for four weeks so that your abdominal muscles have a chance to heal properly. Moderate exercise, such as walking, swimming and cycling are actually beneficial, because they strengthen the muscles without strain and help you to get your figure back. You should avoid driving a motor car for four weeks after the operation; until your abdominal muscles are in good trim, there is a risk that you might not be able to press the brake in time if someone ran in front of the car.

How soon after surgery can you have sex? As soon as you feel comfortable. Some women try for a baby about two weeks after surgery, others find themselves too uncomfortable and bloated to consider sex for three or four weeks. It is possible to conceive within a month of surgery, and we know of many women who did not have a period afterwards for this reason. As far as I am aware, the world record is held by a patient of mine who was found with her husband (a Texan) in a side ward of the hospital by the night nurse making her rounds; this was just three days after a three-hour operation. Her sense of urgency deserved reward, and she conceived.

Follow-up People should be seen at regular intervals after surgery; it is a mistake to feel that you should go away for a year afterwards to 'get on with it'. The better the follow-up, the more chance of success. We like to see couples a minimum of five times, spaced at regular intervals, during the first year after surgery. After that, they are seen every six months. Repeated checks on ovulation and male fertility are made. If you are not pregnant after one year or eighteen months of proper follow-up, a laparoscopy should be discussed with your doctor. Another laparoscopy at this stage will be a much better test than a hysterosalpingogram, because it gives an idea of the amount of adhesion formation – the most common reason for failure of surgery.

How can you prevent another bout of tubal infection after surgery? Unfortunately, this is not always possible, though you can minimize the chances. The following points are worth considering:

1. Report to your gynaecologist if you feel any tenderness in your abdomen or have bouts of pain together with fever or vaginal discharge.
2. Ask your partner to have his semen checked at the time of your operation. A good laboratory will check for bacteria or signs of infection.
3. Avoid tubal x-rays unless you have been prescribed antibiotics (these will fight bacteria that may be introduced that way).

4. If you are unlucky enough to have a miscarriage after surgery
    (sometimes the first pregnancy after tubal surgery does fail by
    miscarriage), make certain that you are given proper antibiotic
    cover to diminish the risk of infection in your tubes.

Should you have your tubes washed through after surgery?   Preferably not. Although it is sometimes still done, this is now regarded
as an obsolete treatment that does no good. It carries an unnecessary risk of introducing bacteria and tends in any case to be rather
painful.

GETTING PREGNANT

This will be your first ambition after a successful operation. There
are a number of questions women frequently ask me:

My friends tell me that I must get pregnant as soon as possible after the surgery, before the adhesions have time to re-form

This is wrong. The process begins within twenty-four hours of
surgery, and almost certainly any adhesions have their roots in the
first forty-eight hours after the operation. You would need to be
very active sexually if you were to beat the adhesion process.
Modern surgical methods are geared to preventing it from starting;
as long as the first few days after surgery are successfully
negotiated, there should be no adhesion development because the
surfaces of the tubes and uterus will have healed. Unless you are
unlucky enough to have another bout of pelvic infection, you will
almost certainly be safe from adhesions.

Will my tubes block again after surgery?

One of the major advantages of microsurgery over the older, more
conventional types of surgery is that tubal blockage is less likely.
Previously, reblockage of the tubes happened in about 45 per cent
of women having an operation. With microsurgery, the risk is less
than 10 per cent. Still, although reblockage is uncommon, this does

not necessarily mean that tubal surgery will succeed; even when the tubes are completely open they may be too damaged to work effectively. This damage may improve only a little after surgery.

Can I get pregnant with only one tube and if so, does this mean that I will be fertile only in alternate months?

It is certainly possible to get pregnant with only one tube – one woman I know has had seven healthy children through one tube, the other having been removed when she was fourteen. Because women do not ovulate from each side in alternate months (it is not true that the right side is for boys and the left for girls!) your fertility may not even be reduced if one tube has been removed. None the less, you are obviously better off with both tubes, and likely to conceive more quickly.

Will I be able to deliver normally after tubal surgery?

Yes, probably. The great majority of women do not have problems at delivery. However, you may be advised to have a Caesarean section after certain types of surgery, particularly the implantation operation. The reason for this is that the operation sometimes leaves the walls of the uterus a little weak.

How long will it take to conceive?

People expect tubal surgery to work immediately. It hardly ever does. Even though your tubes will have been opened perfectly satisfactorily, they will never work entirely normally. An embryo may die because the tubal environment is not perfect, or it may be delayed in transport. For this reason, a number of cycles may be needed before you strike lucky. Think of a woman with damaged tubes as rather like a motor car with only three out of four cylinders firing. It will be likely to reach its destination eventually, but it will take a lot longer than a car that is firing on all four cylinders. So women with more severely damaged tubes tend to take longer to conceive.

After straightforward rejoining operations such as anastomosis, most women who are going to conceive do so in the first eighteen months. It takes longer after unblocking the ovarian end of the tube by salpingostomy, and only about half of the women who have this operation conceive in the first eighteen months. This is probably because the tubes continue to heal for a long time after surgery.

Can tubal surgery be repeated?

Yes, sometimes. At present the success rate of repeat tubal surgery is about the same as for the test-tube baby treatment (see Chapter 10). But some types of tubal damage are really not suitable for a second shot at surgery, particularly if you have a great deal of scarring of your tubal wall or if your tubes are blocked in several places.

Tubal surgery has the best chance of being successful at the first attempt, which is one reason why you should seek referral to a centre doing a good deal of this kind of surgery.

If the surgery fails, would artificial insemination help me?

This is not a treatment for damaged or blocked tubes. Artificial insemination (which you should not confuse with in vitro fertilization – see Chapter 10) does not bypass the tubes. Artificial insemination is done simply by placing semen in the vagina or cervix as a substitute for normal intercourse (see Chapter 9).

Despite the disadvantages I list earlier in this chapter, many women want to try in vitro fertilization because they think tubal surgery has failed. Your decision must depend on the advice you get from your surgeon and the way you and your partner feel about it. Obviously, if you are already over thirty-five, an attempt at test-tube baby treatment might be worth considering soon. If it fails, you still have a chance of getting pregnant if your tubes have been opened successfully. However, the pressures are always great, and the natural tendency is to want to try for a test-tube baby before giving surgery a proper chance of success. We can recall many women who panicked after surgery, went for in vitro fertilization which failed and later had a normal conception. Going for in vitro fertilization too soon can certainly put people under a lot of strain.

We recommend you not to try it until you have had at least one year of normal intercourse after surgery. We make an exception if, for example, during tubal surgery we discover that a woman's tubes are more damaged than we expected.

ENDOMETRIOSIS

This is a disease that is particularly common in the United States and Europe. It is a peculiar condition, where the lining of the uterus, the endometrium, grows not only in its normal place but also in other sites, for example, around the ovaries, the tubes or the outer lining of the pelvic organs (see the diagram on page 76). This may damage the tubes by causing adhesions around them or by scarring them. It can also cause complete tubal blockage, although that is unlikely. Nevertheless, it is a benign disease, in no way similar to cancer, and as it is controlled like your periods by hormones, it disappears at the menopause. It is never life-threatening.

Although it is not usually a direct cause of infertility, I believe it is important to explain endometriosis here and go into some detail about the treatment. Many women coming to my clinic for a laparoscopy are found to have endometriosis. They are particularly worried that this may be linked with their infertility. But as far as we know, anyone may have the same condition and be fertile. A mild case of endometriosis would be discovered only during an investigation for another condition.

Endometriosis may involve the uterine wall (see the diagram on page 76), when it is known as adenomyosis. The uterus becomes enlarged and sometimes tender. Periods tend to be heavy and less regular, and women with adenomyosis are often infertile. There is more information about this condition and its treatment in Chapter 5.

The majority of women with endometriosis are fertile and conceive perfectly normally. However, in some women endometriosis is associated with infertility. When it is very extensive and there are a lot of adhesions and scarring, it is understandable that you may be infertile. The effect on your anatomy alone accounts for the tube failing to pick up an egg. But mostly scarring is very slight and the tubes are open; so some doctors think that it may be infertility that causes endometriosis rather than the other way round.

The precise cause of endometriosis surprisingly remains a mystery, although there are so many theories. The commonest explanation is that endometrial cells, shed at the time of menstruation, do not all travel into the vagina with the menstrual blood, but some flow up the tubes and into the abdominal cavity. Here they may implant and grow into little islands. This explanation is not entirely satisfactory, because most normal women lose some endometrial cells into their tubes during their periods and yet they don't all get endometriosis. Moreover, you would expect endometriosis of the vagina to be very common if this theory were true since the menstrual cells are mostly lost through the vagina. But this is very rare. Another suggestion is that endometrial cells just develop in abnormal sites in some women, but this is hardly satisfactory either.

What are the theories supporting endometriosis as a cause of infertility?

- Interference with ovulation. Some women who have endometriosis do not ovulate regularly. The follicle containing the egg does not burst and the egg cannot leave the ovary. This is thought to be due to chemical interference with ovarian function.
- It is thought endometriosis may produce chemicals that interfere with the normal action of the muscles of the tubes. These chemicals are called prostaglandins, and women with endometriosis seem to have an excess of them. The theory is that the prostaglandins prevent the muscles transporting the embryo into the uterus.
- Excessive prostaglandins may just possibly also prevent the embryo from implanting in the uterus and forming a foetus. Any embryo that is formed is absorbed and lost into the outside world.

What are the symptoms?

Endometriosis may be suspected if you suffer from painful periods or intercourse, or heavy or irregular periods. Obviously many perfectly normal women suffer from heavy irregular periods which

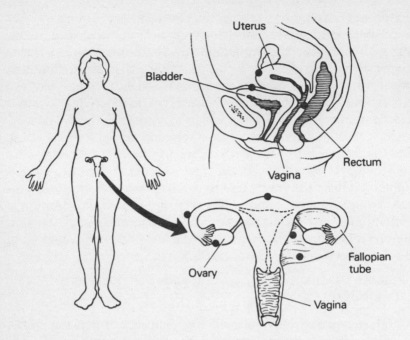

Endometriosis – the shaded areas show where it may grow

are painful, so there generally need to be additional reasons for suspicion. For example, your gynaecologist may think of endometriosis because he can feel lumps or thickening of the tissues when he examines you internally. However, the only definite way to diagnose the disease is to see it. This means having a laparoscopy. Sometimes adhesions are found. If there is any doubt about the diagnosis, your gynaecologist may take a little piece of tissue during the laparoscopy to examine under the microscope. If laparoscopy is offered to you, it is worth having it done sooner rather than later so that any endometriosis is treated promptly.

What are the treatments for endometriosis?

Nothing at all   Endometriosis that is very mild or causing no symptoms carries no risk for you. Because there is considerable doubt as to whether infertility is really caused by endometriosis, many doctors will decide to do nothing. If this is the decision in your case, you might try to maximize your chance of pregnancy by every other method. This could include measures to improve a low sperm count and encouraging ovulation with drugs such as clomiphene (see page 44). Your specialist may also suggest repeating your laparoscopy a year or two after the first diagnosis to see whether the endometriosis has got any worse and needs more active treatment.

Drugs The islands of endometriosis are under the same control by your hormones as the lining of the uterus, or uterus. Just as it is possible to stop your periods with hormone therapy, so it is possible to reduce endometriosis. Drug treatment allows the endometriosis to 'dry up' and heal. Although it is effective in suppressing endometriosis, the islands sometimes grow again when the drugs are stopped. The drugs used are:

* The contraceptive pill; the pill may be given for five or six months. This effectively reduces bleeding and pain. Obviously, while you are taking the pill you cannot get pregnant, so the plan is to reduce the extent of the endometriosis in the hope that you will conceive as soon as the pill is stopped.
  Because pregnancy produces a lot of the same hormones that are given to help endometriosis and during pregnancy you will not menstruate, pregnancy itself is a very effective way of curing endometriosis.
* Progesterone treatment; sufficient amounts of progesterone suppress endometrial growth. Because pure progesterone is expensive and has to be given by injection, doctors usually prescribe synthetic progesterone tablets – normally for about five or six months.
* Danazol treatment; danazol is a synthetically produced by-product of the male hormone, testosterone. It reduces endometrial growth very effectively, but has the disadvantage that it also suppresses your pituitary gland and therefore ovarian activity. Danazol is claimed to dry up endometriosis more effectively than the pill or progesterone. By stopping your ovaries working normally it induces a temporary menopause and, of course, during the menopause endometriosis stops growing completely.

The disadvantage of all these drugs is twofold. First, they all suppress your normal hormones and prevent ovulation. This means you cannot get pregnant while you are taking them. If you don't get pregnant fairly soon after stopping them, you may be back to square one. This is clearly a major problem for older women, who may have only a little time left to conceive. For this reason, I am reluctant to give these drugs at all to women over thirty-five.

Second, all of them can cause side effects. About 20 per cent of women who have drug treatment for endometriosis experience unpleasant effects, such as weight gain, feeling unwell, occasional nausea (at least at the beginning); and some women get a light continuous vaginal discharge which contains blood. Danazol may cause hair loss or excessive hair growth. Because it causes a temporary menopause, a few women get hot flushes, loss of breast tissues and a dry vagina during intercourse. These symptoms all stop entirely when you finish taking the tablets, but they are sufficiently alarming or unpleasant to make some people pull out of treatment early. None the less, if they are recommended, it is certainly worth trying them.

Surgery   Another way is to remove the islands of endometriosis. As mentioned, small islands can sometimes be removed during laparoscopy. The surgeon first inserts a fine metal electrode into the abdomen. Using the telescope to manoeuvre the electrode on to the islands, he or she then passes an electrical current through them and burns them. About 40 per cent of women may conceive after this minor surgery but it is not clear whether they could have conceived without such treatment.

If you have many adhesions or extensive endometriosis, this treatment is not much use. You may be advised to have an open operation. This means fairly major surgery and the procedure and its effects are similar to tubal surgery (see page 64).

Open surgery for endometriosis is best done in centres where there are proper facilities for microsurgery. The islands of endometriosis can be cut away, adhesions divided and any blood-filled cysts on the ovary removed. The surgery is technically difficult and demands great experience for the best results. But it is not at all dangerous and after effects are exceptionally rare. Unfortunately, because the adhesions caused by endometriosis are often very extensive, it is not always possible to remove them all or to get a complete cure. The chances of a pregnancy with an experienced surgeon are good and about 60 per cent of women conceive within a year, provided there are no other problems causing infertility. One big advantage of surgery is that, unlike drug treatment, you can try for a baby within two or three weeks of the operation. This is why surgery is often the better option for older women.

In vitro fertilization   If the adhesions due to endometriosis cannot be entirely removed, in vitro fertilization may be suggested.

Many women with endometriosis fear that they may end up having a hysterectomy. In fact, the only reason for hysterectomy would be if you had very severe pain indeed. In the vast majority of cases pain can be well controlled by drugs and radical surgery is hardly ever advised if you are infertile. Remember that endometriosis tends to disappear when you get beyond forty, and so the threat of hysterectomy is an unnecessary worry.

What are the long term results?

I am often asked by women who have had surgery for endometriosis whether the condition will return if they don't get pregnant quickly. Surgery, effectively done, offers a permanent cure for at least 60 per cent of patients. This means that chances of conception are not reduced for a year or even longer after surgery. However, because endometriosis is not always completely eradicated, you should consider having a laparoscopy about a year after the operation if you haven't conceived.

If you do get pregnant, don't worry about the endometriosis affecting the pregnancy or the baby. Even bad scarring or adhesions have remarkably little effect on a pregnancy and the fact that you have had endometriosis does not increase the risk of a miscarriage, an ectopic pregnancy or a difficult delivery. There is no added risk of an abnormality affecting your baby.

5

Uterine problems

Infertility due to problems of the uterus is a little different. Quite frequently, women who have a uterine abnormality have no difficulty in actually getting pregnant. Their problem is often that they have great trouble keeping a pregnancy, as they tend to miscarry in the first months after conception.

Although uterine problems causing infertility are not common (only about 5 to 10 per cent of female infertility), they are important because they are sometimes overlooked. They can really be divided into two categories. The first is where there is an abnormality of the upper part of the uterus, or uterine body (see the diagram on page 83). The second is an abnormality of the neck of the uterus, or cervix. Problems with the cervix are equally infrequent, and hardly ever cause symptoms.

WHAT ARE THE CAUSES?

Diseases of the uterine body

Many women have a problem without being infertile. Nevertheless, these conditions can lead to infertility:

Fibroids These are benign growths of muscle, which appear in the wall of the uterus. They are virtually never malignant and are

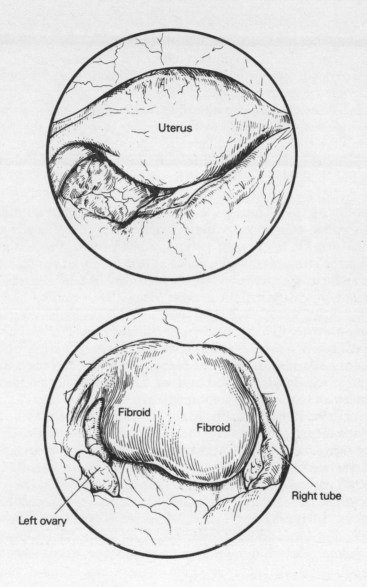

ABOVE, *a normal shaped uterus seen from above and,* BELOW, *extensive fibroid growth*

among the commonest tumours known; it has been calculated that
by the age of forty about one third of British and American women
have some fibroids in their uterus. The majority are not even
detected, but some women have abnormal periods and a few in the
younger age group become infertile.

It is not clear how the infertility is caused, but it seems that the
fibroids may distort the uterine cavity and prevent the embryo
implanting. Occasionally, fibroids protruding from the outside of
the uterus seem to cause infertility by displacing the tubes and
ovaries, possibly interfering with transport of the egg.

Uterine polyps   These are smaller growths than most fibroids and
are pretty common. In most women they don't really cause
problems. Quite often the polyp is a small fibroid that has grown
from the uterine wall and is dangling in the uterine cavity. They can
interfere with conception – probably acting like a foreign body in
the uterine cavity, in the same way as the IUD or coil.

Adenomyosis   This disease is a puzzling one, but it is less common
than fibroids. Probably about 10 to 15 per cent of uterine problems
causing infertility are due to adenomyosis. It is similar to endometriosis (see Chapter 4) and, indeed, can go together with it. It is
benign and causes no symptoms. The name adenomyosis is given
to the condition where little islands of the endometrium (the lining
of the uterus) grow outside the uterine cavity, forming pockets in
the uterine wall itself. These cause trouble because at each period
they bleed into themselves, but there is no outlet for the blood
which collects. Scar tissue forms around the islands in the uterine
muscle and so if there are a lot of little pockets, the uterus becomes
enlarged, irregular and tender. Adenomyosis can cause quite severe
period pain and also heavy periods. Why it causes infertility is not
absolutely clear, but the changed uterine shape, the disturbance of
the uterine blood supply and possibly associated chemical changes,
may have something to do with it.

Adhesions in the uterine cavity   Occasionally, the insides of the
walls of the uterus are totally or partially stuck together. Intrauterine adhesions (or synechiae) usually follow a surgical injury of
some kind, such as over-vigorous scraping of the uterus after an

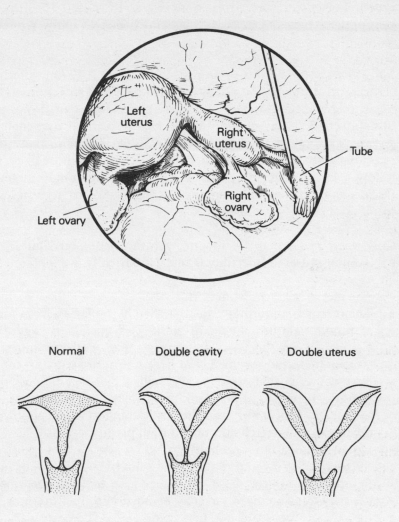

Left
uterus

Right
uterus

Tube

Right
ovary

Left ovary

Normal   Double cavity   Double uterus

ABOVE, *a double uterus, the left side better developed and more normal;* BELOW, *diagrammatic representation of the normal uterus compared with unusual developments* abortion or miscarriage. Adhesions can also be caused by tuberculosis of the uterus, but this is an uncommon disease in the Western world.

Inflammation of the uterine lining   Wearing an IUD (intrauterine contraceptive device) or possibly some bacterial infections may cause inflammation inside the uterus. Tuberculosis can also cause this. Infection, however, is not likely to be caused by venereal disease, as some women fear. As far as we know, intrauterine infection is not caused by sexual contact. It is much more likely to follow a failed pregnancy, trouble with a coil or minor surgery. Occasionally, chronic inflammation in the uterine cavity can lead to adhesions in it (see above).

Congenital problems   These are problems from birth and are uncommon causes of infertility. There are basically five types:

- The uterus is absent from birth.
- The uterus is abnormally small (called hypoplasia); from time to time an abnormally small uterus is a mistaken diagnosis. Congenital smallness is extremely rare. Perfectly normal women (especially women who have not been pregnant) often have a uterus that seems very small. This does not usually indicate a congenital problem or a failure of development. In literally 95 per cent of cases there is nothing to worry about, as the uterus will stretch normally during pregnancy.
- Double uterus: during a baby girl's first few months of life in the uterus, her own uterus develops from two tubes, or cornua. Before she is born, these two tubes fuse to form the single uterus. Occasionally, a girl may be born with two uteruses, if the uterine tubes did not fuse completely. There are various degrees of failure to fuse, and most of them cause absolutely no problem in adult life. A few may cause a tendency to miscarry and sometimes failure to conceive. A double uterus by no means always causes infertility. One woman aged forty who I delivered had twins, with a boy in one uterus and a girl in the other.
- The T-shaped uterus: this is another defect of uterine fusion which has received some attention in the press. It happened to

some girls whose mothers were given a particular hormone therapy, diethylstilboestrol, during early pregnancy. Ironically, these hormones used to be given to help women who were prone to lose their babies in the first few months of pregnancy. They had the unfortunate side effect of causing uterine abnormalities in some of the babies. This condition is rare in Britain but is slightly more common in the USA, where this drug treatment was popular in the 1950s.

• Asymmetrical development of the uterus. Sometimes one uterine tube develops more than the other, making a unicornate uterus. Some women with this problem are infertile or more likely to miscarry. Women with a unicornate uterus are also prone to ectopic pregnancy.

Is a tilted uterus a cause of infertility? This is a question that worries enormous numbers of women. A great many women have a uterus that is tilted either to one side or backwards (the medical name is retroverted). This used to be considered a possible cause of infertility. Actually, almost 25 per cent of women have a retroverted uterus, and it may reassure you to know that 25 per cent of women attending antenatal clinics have a retroverted uterus at the start of pregnancy. As the baby grows the position is rectified. Retroversion may be connected with infertility only if you have a related problem, such as severe adhesions, and this will be discovered in your routine checks.

WHAT ARE THE SYMPTOMS?

There are often no symptoms to indicate that the uterus is the cause of your infertility. However, if you have any of the following, your doctor may suspect uterine disease:

No periods   A few women with fairly severe uterine disease have no periods at all. Obviously, there are many causes for this symptom, and a common one is some form of ovarian failure (see Chapter 3). Loss of periods due to uterine problems can mean that the uterus is completely absent or, more likely, there is scar tissue replacing the normal uterine lining (or endometrium).

Scanty or infrequent periods   This symptom, like the previous one, is likely to be due to a problem with the ovaries. However, a few women with a uterine problem may have scanty periods (oligomenorrhoea) because of scar tissue in the uterine lining, or because of an infection.

Heavy periods   These may be due to fibroids or adenomyosis. They can also be caused by an infection in the uterus. The commonest cause is hormonal.

Painful periods (dysmenorrhoea) are, of course, extremely common, and seldom associated with a uterine problem. The majority of women with dysmenorrhoea are absolutely normal. However, painful periods are occasionally caused by a polyp, fibroids or adenomyosis.

Bleeding between periods   Only a tiny fraction of women with bleeding between periods have uterine disease, such as fibroids, as the cause of their infertility. But it is an important symptom of other diseases, and if you have this bleeding it is always advisable to talk to your doctor about it.

Repeated miscarriages   Some women manage to get pregnant but every time they conceive, they lose the pregnancy, for the reasons described in Chapter 7.

WHAT ARE THE SPECIAL TESTS FOR UTERINE PROBLEMS?

There are several ways that uterine abnormalities may be detected by your doctor. If an abnormality is suspected, more than one test is usually needed.

1. Simple physical examination. Fibroids, when they are fairly large, can be detected just by feeling the abdomen. A pelvic examination, when your doctor examines you internally, may pick up a minor enlargement of the uterus and some congenital abnormalities are found this way.

2. Dilatation and curettage (D and C). This small operation, widely performed for a great many gynaecological problems, requires a quick anaesthetic. It is not painful afterwards. The cervix is first dilated (hence 'dilatation') to allow an instrument into the uterine cavity. Next, the uterine lining is scraped (hence 'curettage'). D and C is of limited use for detecting infertility, but it can be used to discover fibroids or polyps. During a D and C, it is usual to take a piece of the uterine lining (an endometrial biopsy, see page 42) so that it can be examined for other conditions as well. This is essential if, for example, tuberculosis is suspected.

3. X-ray (hysterosalpingogram). One of the most useful tests is a hysterosalpingogram when dye, which shows up on an x-ray photograph, is gently injected into the uterus (for a fuller description of this test, see page 58). The cavity of the uterus is outlined and irregularities, often caused by fibroids, adeno-myosis or polyps, may be detected. Congenital abnormalities of the uterus can usually be very accurately diagnosed – for example, a double uterus will show up as two distinct shadows on the photograph. Adhesions and tuberculosis can also be detected on the x-ray.

4. Laparoscopy (see Chapter 3). If you have an infection or a uterine abnormality shows on an x-ray, your doctor will want to inspect the outside of your uterus. As x-rays show only the inside, laparoscopy may be necessary to see if the outside of the uterus is abnormal as well.

5. Ultrasound (see Chapter 3). If a uterine problem is suspected to be causing infertility, ultrasound can be used to see if your uterine cavity is irregular and if there is a congenital defect. Since many hospitals are not properly equipped for testing fertility by ultrasound, you may be glad to know it is certainly not essential for discovering uterine problems.

6. Hysteroscopy. This is the inspection of the uterine cavity with a telescope, or hysteroscope. The instrument is about the thickness of a pencil and is inserted through the cervix. This usually requires an anaesthetic and may mean an overnight stay in the hospital. Some doctors do it on an outpatient basis. There is no pain afterwards, but a few women have a little vaginal bleeding. Hysteroscopy is not dangerous. Its advantage

is that it gives your doctor a direct view of the uterine cavity and it can be used to detect abnormalities of shape. It is particularly useful for seeing adhesions in the uterus and can even be used for treating them. The hysteroscope can be used to position other instruments, such as tiny scissors, inside the uterus to divide adhesions or remove polyps. Using it is still rather specialized and though this test is very convenient, it is not available everywhere. Fortunately, it can often be replaced by more conventional tests.

7. Post-coital tests. These I describe in Chapter 6.

TREATMENTS

These are mainly straightforward and successful; for example, around 55 per cent of women we treat get pregnant within a year of having fibroids removed.

The uterine body

Fibroids normally do not need any treatment. If your doctor is certain that the fibroids are causing infertility or repeated miscarriages, removing them may be recommended. This operation, called myomectomy, is not dangerous, but it means you have to spend at least a week in hospital. As far as preparation and after care are concerned the operation is similar to tubal surgery (see Chapter 4).

Just occasionally, fibroids are big enough to need a hysterectomy, and yet the woman concerned would desperately like to get pregnant. It is difficult to give open and shut advice in this case. Obviously, if you have a large mass in the abdomen, there is always the faint suspicion that it may not be due to fibroids but something else. If the lump is symptomless, your doctor may have suggested hysterectomy just to be on the safe side. Obviously, no doctor can give categorical assurances about the nature of a lump until it is removed. A laparoscopy may be worth considering and, if combined with a D and C, may help confirm the diagnosis. You must bear in mind that even if you decide to have just the fibroids removed by a myomectomy, this may not be satisfactory. This is

true if you have very large fibroids, or a great many. A big
myomectomy seldom results in a pregnancy and there is always the
faint chance that you may develop more fibroids later and need to
return for a hysterectomy. The best thing to do is to have a very
thorough discussion with your doctor.

Polyps Treatment is simple in most cases; removing them needs
only a quick anaesthetic. The operation is essentially a curettage,
and means spending a night at most in hospital.

Adenomyosis Treatment in the early stages is usually by drugs.
There are several hormone preparations that reduce the menstrual
flow. When taken by women with adenomyosis, they tend to cut
down the bleeding into the uterine muscle.

While you are on hormones for adenomyosis, your periods may
stop completely. Actually this is the best treatment, because the
scar tissue occurs around the bleeding islands at period time. You
will not get pregnant on the pills, but when you stop them there is
an increased possibility of your conceiving. The chance of the
adenomyosis returning after you've finished treatment is not too
high. It is very slow-growing, and there is usually plenty of time to
get pregnant first. Getting pregnant is the best treatment of all, as
pregnancy itself provides the very hormones that stop you menstruating.

Women with more advanced adenomyosis may need surgery.
The operation is very similar to myomectomy and is not risky. If
the adenomyosis is very extensive and causing severe pain, then
your doctor may suggest a hysterectomy. This, though, is hardly
ever necessary.

Adhesions Treatment is geared to division of the adhesions,
which is a minor surgical procedure (rather like a D and C)
requiring an overnight stay in hospital. This may be done using a
hysteroscope, the telescope inserted in the uterus. The surgeon may
decide to place an IUD in the uterus for a month after division. This
keeps the walls of the uterus apart during healing and prevents
further adhesions from forming. You will be given antibiotics at
the same time to diminish the chance of infection, hormones to
promote good growth and a new uterine lining, and possibly

steroids to reduce further adhesion formation. Treatment is not always immediately successful, so repeated attempts to divide the adhesions may be necessary. You shouldn't worry about having repeated treatments too much. They are rather like chipping away at a rock – doing a little bit more each time.

Tuberculosis adhesions may not be treatable because the uterine lining cannot grow again.

Inflammation of the uterine lining   If you have inflammation, any foreign body in the uterus such as a forgotten coil will be removed and you will be given a course of antibiotics. This is usually very effective.

Congenital abnormalities   Treatment varies. There is no treatment possible if your uterus has not developed at all. A genuinely small uterus can occasionally be treated with hormone preparations. In fairly exceptional circumstances, surgery may be suggested to correct the other deformities – the medical name for the operation is metroplasty (plastic reconstruction of the uterus). The risks and complications are similar to those for tubal surgery.

PROBLEMS WITH THE CERVIX

Narrowed or scarred cervix

The cervix may be scarred as a result of an injury, perhaps after a difficult delivery or an abortion. Scar tissue causes the cervix to be narrowed. It may also prevent cervical mucus production, so that there may not be enough mucus for the sperm to swim around in. Occasionally the scarring of the cervix is so bad that the cervical canal which runs through it becomes completely blocked. If this happens, menstrual blood will be unable to leave the uterus and will collect in the uterine cavity, which can give rise to infection.

Dilated or incompetent cervix

This does not cause true infertility, but it may result in miscarriages. The cervical canal is wide either from birth or as a result of surgical injury, for example after a vigorous dilatation in a D and C operation (see page 87, or a termination of pregnancy. It occasionally results from a cone biopsy of the cervix. This may have been done to remove precancerous areas in the cervix. The surgeon may need to remove the whole of the lower part of the cervix, so that miscarriage tends to happen after the twelfth week of pregnancy. Repeated miscarriage before this time is unlikely to be due to this condition.

Problems with cervical mucus There is hardly any subject in the field of infertility that confuses people more than this. Because it is such a difficult area for both doctors and the women concerned and because it is so controversial, a separate chapter is devoted to it (see Chapter 6).

What are the symptoms?

Most cervical problems cause none. A scarred or narrowed cervix may occasionally cause painful periods because the menstrual blood cannot escape easily. If the scarring is very severe and your cervix totally blocked, your periods may stop completely, but you would feel severe pain at period time.

A dilated cervix causes no symptoms beyond repeated miscarriage, which will normally be the first and only sign that something is wrong.

Problems with the cervical mucus cause a negative post-coital test (see Chapter 6).

Treatment

Treatment for a narrowed or scarred cervix involves dilatation – a very simple procedure needing a quick general anaesthetic. This may have to be done more than once over several months.

To help healing of a scarred cervical surface, treatment with freezing or a laser may also be suggested. Both these treatments are painless. Yet cervical scarring can be easily overlooked, because

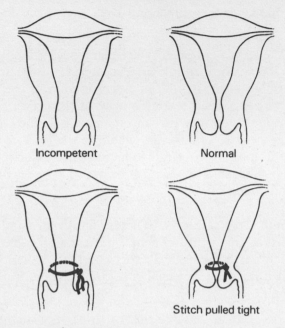

Incompetent   Normal

Stitch pulled tight

The stitch operation for an incompetent cervix

it is unusual. One woman, who was investigated for infertility for seven years, had endless tests and many hormone treatments. Repeated artificial insemination failed to produce a pregnancy and her marital life was in tatters. A simple ten-minute procedure, dilatation of the cervix, resulted in conception within two weeks. She later had two more children without any difficulty.

A dilated cervix   This involves reconstruction of the cervix by surgery, an operation that is simple for the woman but quite difficult to perform accurately. For this reason and because it is just as effective, most surgeons prefer instead to introduce a stitch during pregnancy. At about the twelfth week of pregnancy, a nylon stitch or tape is placed around the outside of the cervix. This keeps it shut during pregnancy. The operation means having a short anaesthetic and a few days rest in hospital. It is painless and modern methods of anaesthesia are completely harmless to the pregnancy. You can expect to see some bloodstained discharge after cervical stitching; this is likely to last up to two weeks at least.

It is nothing to worry about and does not mean that another miscarriage is threatened.

You may think that putting a stitch around the cervix during pregnancy will itself increase the chance of miscarriage. In fact, this is a gentle operation and causes little disturbance. The risks of not having it done greatly outweigh the very faint risk of inducing a miscarriage.

During or just before labour the stitch will be removed. You must not deliver past it, otherwise your cervix may get more damaged. If you go into labour unexpectedly, your doctor will remove it for you then. If you go to term, it is common practice to have the stitch removed at about thirty-eight weeks. This is very simple and can be done painlessly without anaesthetic; normally it requires just a snip. If you decide later to go for a second pregnancy, you may need a stitch again to keep your cervix closed.

One final word about a worry couples often have: if you do get pregnant having been infertile with a uterine problem, your baby has the same chances as any other of being normal. There is no increased risk of having an abnormal baby simply because your uterus is or has been abnormal.

6

Problems with cervical mucus

This must be the most controversial area in infertility. I remember one international meeting where two eminent professors disagreed so strongly about the importance of testing the cervical mucus that they refused to talk to each other for three years afterwards. Some doctors consider cervical mucus problems to be a complete fantasy; others think this is the single most important area of investigation and treatment. The truth almost certainly lies somewhere in between. When trying to discover the cause of a couple's infertility, every avenue should be explored.

The present estimate is that about 5 per cent of female infertility is due to problems with cervical mucus. That means that a substantial number of women have mucus problems. In this chapter we shall look at some of the facts and myths.

WHAT IS CERVICAL MUCUS AND WHAT DOES IT DO?

The cervical mucus is a jelly-like substance produced by tiny glands in the cervical canal, which leads from the vagina into the uterus. The mucus acts effectively like a cork in the cervix and may prevent bacteria getting into the uterine cavity. It changes in chemical composition and consistency during the menstrual cycle. During the first half of the cycle before ovulation, when the hormone estrogen is produced in ever increasing amounts (see Chapter 1), the mucus made by the cervical glands becomes more watery and copious. Large amounts are produced immediately before ovulation. Some women make so much at this time that they can see it as a watery vaginal discharge. Then it can be a pointer in working out the exact day of ovulation, as normally this discharge lasts about twelve to thirty-six hours. Sperm can penetrate the watery mucus, and when intercourse takes place they swim through it into the uterus.

After ovulation the quality of the mucus changes. The ovary now starts to make the hormone progesterone. Mucus produced under progesterone influence is thicker and more sticky; there is also less of it. This mucus is impenetrable to sperm. This is one reason why intercourse after ovulation is not fertile, even though an egg may be waiting in the fallopian tube.

It has been calculated that even when intercourse occurs at the time the cervical mucus is at its most favourable, only about one in every two thousand sperm enter the mucus. The rest stay in the vagina, where they die. This is because the vaginal fluid is naturally acid, which is not suitable for sperm. Those that have entered the mucus can survive there for long periods – certainly for several days after intercourse. Once in the cervical mucus, they steadily escape from it into the uterus over a period of at least seventy-two hours. So the cervical mucus can act as a kind of reservoir, to be called on if intercourse does not take place at the best time.

There are several reasons why it is thought cervical mucus may prevent the sperm moving freely into the uterus:

- There is not enough of it to allow the sperm to move easily
- It is too thick and sticky
- It is not compatible with your partner's sperm.

To decide whether any of these is your problem, your doctor will investigate both of you, an experience that can be rather tiresome. Because this is such a controversial subject, in this chapter I have discussed all the worries my patients raise with me, and I hope to show what is generally agreed among doctors and what is myth.

TESTS ON CERVICAL MUCUS

Problems with cervical mucus usually cause no symptoms. The first test that is routinely done is the post-coital test.

The post-coital test (PCT)   This is one of the oldest tests in investigating infertility and has been done for well over a hundred years. What happens is very simple. The gynaecologist examines a small sample of your cervical mucus under a microscope some hours after sexual intercourse. The mucus is sucked painlessly from the cervical canal during an internal examination. Most doctors feel that the best time to do this is about six to twenty-four hours after sex, but this timing is not that critical. If the test is positive – that is, normal – live sperm will be seen swimming in the mucus sample. Theoretically, the sperm should be swimming in a fairly straight line and reasonably vigorously. If the sperm are swimming straight this suggests that your mucus is of the right chemical composition.

In a negative test the sperm are seen swimming around very slowly in all directions, or none are seen at all, or they are all dead. If this happens at the first test, the doctor will probably want you to do several PCTs over a period of time as the test can be negative initially even though your mucus is normal (see below).

Ferning   Another test which is done occasionally is the 'ferning' test. This is to see whether your hormones are normal after ovulation (see also Chapter 3). A small drop of mucus is placed on a glass slide and allowed to dry. It should crystallize, forming branches which look very like fern leaves. The amount of branching depends on the influence of estrogen and progesterone, and so this test can be used also to see if your mucus is responding normally to hormones. If the mucus seems to be abnormal, a test using a dried specimen of your mucus under very high magnification (up to x 10,000) with a specialized electron microscope may be done. At this power, the minute details of its composition can be seen.

If your PCT is positive it implies that:

1. Your partner is likely to be producing enough normal sperm
2. There is nothing wrong with intercourse
3. You are producing sufficient normal hormones before ovulation and it is not so likely that you have a problem with ovulation
4. There are no antibodies in your mucus hostile to the sperm (see page 98).

If your PCT is negative this does not necessarily mean you are killing your partner's sperm. A great many women are worried that they are doing this, and yet there are many other reasons why no sperm, or only dead sperm, are seen in the post-coital test. Most are unconnected with infertility. In our clinic, 85 per cent of women who have a negative test are perfectly normal and so are their partners. A negative test is meaningful only if it is repeatedly negative under perfect conditions. Some of the reasons for a negative test are:

- *Your PCT was not done at the best time* – for example, you might have ovulated early that month, and so the mucus came under the influence of progesterone rather than estrogen. Alternatively, the PCT may have been done too early in the cycle, before your mucus had a chance to get really watery and be receptive to sperm. Wrong timing is the commonest reason for a negative test, and can even cause repeatedly negative tests.
- *You just didn't ovulate the month of the test* – perhaps because of the strain or stress of making love to order. Consequently, you didn't produce enough estrogen to make good mucus. Failure to ovulate in a particular month is extremely common in perfectly normal women.
- *You may not be ovulating* and so you are not producing enough estrogen. Hormone tests will be needed (see Chapter 3).
- *You partner just didn't produce good semen* when you had intercourse. This, in itself, does not mean there is anything wrong with him, but sperm counts will be needed. Obviously, men with persistently low sperm counts, or men with poorly motile sperm, may be responsible for a negative PCT (see Chapter 9).

- *There may be an abnormality of your cervix* (see also Chapter 5) Bad infection in the cervix may prevent production of adequate mucus. So may damaged gland cells. Some women with a scarred cervix may not produce enough mucus, or possibly mucus of the right type. These problems, though uncommon, are usually easy to treat.
- *Your cervix is producing antibodies to the sperm* Antibodies normally protect the body from invasion by foreign substances (or antigens), especially bacteria. It is these antibodies that prevent us getting infected with, say, whooping cough, after immunization. After sperm have entered the woman's body, the cervix especially may become 'immunized' or 'sensitized' against them so that they are seen as foreign substances and destroyed by specially produced antibodies. Your partner can even make antibodies against his own sperm, which end up being killed. These two problems are not nearly as common as people believe.

  How do you find out if there are any sperm antibodies? Your specialist may want to mix some of your mucus with healthy sperm from a donor. This is done under a microscope. He or she may also suggest mixing some of your partner's sperm with healthy mucus from a donor – also under a microscope. If your partner's sperm don't penetrate that, there could be a problem with the sperm.

  There are also special tests that can be done on a semen or a blood sample, which can detect certain antibodies.
- *There may be a sexual problem* – that is to say, ejaculation may not be taking place inside the vagina. This is a very rare cause of infertility but easy to check (see Chapter 9).
- *You may be taking hormone pills* that are having a bad effect on your mucus. Clomid (clomiphene), tamoxifen, progesterones and Danol (danazol) – all drugs used for infertility problems – can have this effect. One of the reasons that clomiphene, prescribed to help you ovulate, is given early in the cycle is so that it does not interfere with the production of good mucus later on in mid-cycle; even so, it can occasionally give rise to problems. Ask your doctor about this.

If you have had repeatedly negative PCTs, the following conditions should be used to confirm one way or the other whether your mucus is normal:

1. Make certain that the timing of the test is absolutely right before or around, but not after ovulation
2. Have the doctor confirm that you are ovulating, by giving you hormone tests in the cycle being tested
3. Ask your doctor whether your cervix feels normal
4. Confirm that your partner is producing good semen by getting him tested
5. Make sure that intercourse is normal
6. Any cervical infection may need to be treated with antibiotics. If you have bad infection of the cervix your doctor may need to cauterize or freeze your cervix a few weeks before repeating the PCT. These are minor treatments and can be done quickly during an outpatient visit.

By this time you may feel another post-coital test is more than you can bear. Many people find it very unpleasant because they have difficulty performing sex 'to order'. You have my sympathy. One of the major problems about infertility tests, and particularly the post-coital test, is that there is a colossal interference with your sex life. Keep cool. Bear in mind that this is one of the commonest difficulties couples face – some men even become impotent and can't get an erection in these circumstances. Whatever you do, don't let this be a source of conflict between the two of you. The post-coital test can wait – it mostly is not that important anyway; it's a test that has been greatly overemphasized by both doctors and patients. Remember that all infertility specialists have known women who conceived eventually without treatment, even though every post-coital test was negative.

TREATMENT

What do you do if the tests finally confirm your mucus is the problem? This is one area where so many myths flourish. Unfortunately some of the remedies people want to try have no effect on abnormal mucus.

I'm told that some people kill the sperm because of acidity. Would douches to correct this help me?

All women have acid in the vagina. This is protective and prevents infection. The vagina itself is indeed hostile to sperm – left there, they die in any woman. This does not affect fertility, because enough sperm enter the cervix where they are protected against the acid vagina. Although many women have been prescribed douches of various sorts – douches of bicarbonate are a popular choice – there is absolutely no evidence that they are necessary or helpful.

Cervical mucus is produced when there is a lot of estrogen in the body. Will estrogen tablets or vaginal cream make my post-coital test positive?

This is true only up to a point. Although estrogen is sometimes prescribed (often in the form of stilboestrol or Premarin – two popular drugs), there is only slight evidence to suggest that this will help you get pregnant.

All that the estrogens do is to help the cervix produce a great deal of watery mucus. However, estrogens given in most doses are contraceptive (hence their use in the contraceptive pill). If estrogens have produced a positive post-coital test in your case, this may mean that you are not ovulating normally and therefore not producing enough of your own estrogen. Then the correct treatment generally is to take pills to help ovulation rather than to improve your mucus.

Some pills, especially Clomid, are called anti-estrogens – that is, although they induce ovulation, they prevent the cervix producing enough mucus. If that is your problem, you may need to take less Clomid or take it earlier in your cycle. It may even be a good idea to take Clomid and estrogen in the same cycle. Your doctor will be able to advise you about this.

After intercourse, most of the sperm seem to run out of my vagina. Isn't this why my post-coital test is negative?

Loss of seminal fluid after intercourse is perfectly normal, and most women notice some discharge immediately after sex. Many infertile couples imagine that this is the cause of their problem. If your partner had his climax inside you, then you can be sure that no matter how much fluid you lose afterwards, enough sperm will reach the cervical mucus. This discharge is not a cause of infertility.

I've been told that I produce antibodies that are killing the sperm. Can anything be done?

Yes. For this condition the outlook is now more hopeful:

- Some doctors recommend that you avoid contact with sperm for a period of time and then the antibodies may disappear. This is because they are not being stimulated by repeated exposure to the antigen – in this case the sperm. This does not mean that you shouldn't have sex, but when you do your partner should wear a condom so that the sperm don't come into contact with your cervix and vagina. This course may be recommended for six months, until the antibodies have disappeared. This treatment is rarely suggested nowadays because, obviously, if you have intercourse while your partner is wearing a condom, you cannot get pregnant. Most doctors feel that this treatment is something of a gamble. It certainly throws a considerable strain on a couple. I feel that using a condom is not worth trying.
- Some doctors have tried insemination with the husband's semen directly into the uterus. This means bypassing the cervix and therefore the site of the antibodies. It is done by placing a little tube through the cervix into the uterus and injecting a small quantity of treated sperm from your partner through the tube. This treatment has had limited success in some clinics but there is doubt about its value. This is because if you are producing antibodies, the antibodies may be in the fallopian tube and the uterine cavity as well.
- Drugs may be given to prevent you producing antibodies. These act just like the drugs that are given after a kidney transplant to prevent rejection – such as corticosteroids. To be effective they have to be given in quite high doses, and this may cause side effects such as decreased resistance to infection, fluid retention and making you feel rather unwell. Sometimes

intermittent treatment during the first half of the menstrual cycle only is suggested, as this reduces unwanted side effects. However, these treatments are rather experimental and not definitely effective, so you will need to discuss them carefully with your doctor first.

- The test-tube baby treatment: we now know for certain that, even if you have antibodies, they don't prevent fertilization outside your body. For this reason, in vitro fertilization may be the best treatment for this problem. Certainly a small number of women have already been helped by this when antibodies have been the only problem.

There is every reason for investigating the possibility of cervical mucus problems, but it should be done with you and your partner's agreement and alongside tests for other causes of your infertility. It is important that tensions over the PCT are reduced. If you find that an attempt at timed intercourse for a PCT doesn't work out, don't worry. This happens to nearly all couples at some point and it is never as important as it seems at the time.

7

Miscarriage and ectopic pregnancy

To miscarry is one of the most depressing events imaginable. Although the prime effect is on the woman, the man too has to cope with the loss. It is one of nature's evil ironies that infertile women are much more prone to miscarry than other women. If you have been trying for a baby for years and you finally succeed only to miscarry, you feel you've reached the point of despair. As many as 10 to 15 per cent of all pregnancies end with a miscarriage, and it may be some consolation to know that so many pregnancies miscarry. At least it can help you to realize that many other women find themselves in the same boat before finally having a baby. In this chapter I hope to give you some idea of your chances of success another time, and the best ways of maximizing them.

Certain kinds of treatment seem to have a somewhat higher risk of miscarriage: treatments for uterine disease, ovulatory problems and tubal surgery and the test-tube baby technique. Some women who are perfectly fertile in every other way just keep losing the pregnancy soon after conceiving. This in itself is a form of subfertility, and is the reason for about 5 per cent of all cases of infertility.

The medical term for miscarriage, that is losing your baby before the twenty-eighth week of pregnancy, is abortion. The word abortion is usually thought to mean deliberately terminating a pregnancy, but your doctor's use of it does not imply anything sinister. Women who have repeated miscarriages are often said to have 'habitual abortions'. Most miscarriages occur between six to twelve weeks after the date of your last period.

You will be reassured to know that the further you get into pregnancy, the less likely you are to lose the baby.

A few miscarriages, probably about 15 per cent, happen after the twelfth week of pregnancy. These tend to have a different cause and are much more disturbing because by this time you are actively planning for your baby. Worse still, late miscarriages (so-called second-trimester or late abortions) usually produce more bleeding and labour pains, which may be very debilitating.

How do you know if you are miscarrying?

Miscarriage usually starts with a little bleeding or cramps like period pains. If you have these symptoms and you are pregnant, you should speak to your doctor immediately. This is especially true if you have had difficulty getting pregnant.

If you're pregnant and start having any vaginal bleeding at all it really is important that you go to see your doctor immediately. This could herald a miscarriage which may be prevented by rest.

Any unexplained colicky pain, such as the cramps some women feel during a period, can also be early signs of a miscarriage threatening and it is wise to seek advice. However, you need not be unduly alarmed. It is not unusual to have lower abdominal discomfort during pregnancy, and mostly this does not have any kind of serious cause.

WHAT CAUSES MISCARRIAGE?

Often this is just not known. There seems no reason for most miscarriages, and why they should be so common is a mystery. If you miscarry repeatedly, the best way to prevent it happening next time is to try to find the cause. It may be any of the following:

Genetic Sometimes a defective embryo is formed. One in a hundred babies are born with a chromosomal defect, but this is much more common in miscarried pregnancies. Chromosomes carry the unique messages which dictate each individual's characteristics. Occasionally the chromosomes are abnormal, so that an abnormal message can result in an abnormal foetus being formed. At least 30 per cent of abortions have chromosomal defects; miscarriage is nature's safety valve, preventing abnormal babies from surviving a full pregnancy. Very occasionally, repeated miscarriage occurs because one or both of the parents have a chromosomal abnormality and this may be passed on to the foetus. Chromosomal abnormalities do not always show up, and the parents may be entirely normal in every other way. Yet when the defective chromosome is inherited in the embryo, it can be 'expressed' and a defect occurs. If the defect is incompatible with normal life, a miscarriage is likely.

Hormonal You may miscarry because you are not producing enough of the right hormones, or because you have too much male hormone. The foetus may not then implant properly in your uterus.

Some women seem not to produce enough progesterone, the hormone that comes from the ovary after ovulation. This is to help uterine growth and the embryo until the pregnancy itself can make enough progesterone. Some doctors believe that low progesterone production may encourage miscarriage. This theory is doubtful.

There is now definite evidence that a substantial number of women who have abnormalities of LH production are much more likely to miscarry. The commonest cause of this abnormality is polycystic ovarian disease (see page 50). Repeated blood tests in the beginning of the menstrual cycle will reveal whether or not your LH is raised. If it is, then treatment for polycystic ovarian disease is likely to help. One treatment currently being used is suppression of the LH hormone level by giving GnRH treatment (page 48).

Uterine If your uterus is misshapen, perhaps because of fibroids or a minor congenital abnormality (see Chapter 5), it may not be able to support a growing pregnancy and so you can miscarry. These miscarriages tend to happen later in pregnancy rather than in the first three months. Fortunately, with each pregnancy the risk of miscarriage is reduced as the uterine shape changes.

Cervical   Occasionally, the cervical canal may be open (this is called cervical incompetence). This many cause premature labour or miscarriage after the twelfth week of pregnancy (see Chapter 5).

Infections   Certain germs or bacteria may cause a miscarriage. Exactly which bacteria do this is the subject of a lot of argument. They include:

* Brucella – definitely causes miscarriages in cattle
* Toxoplasmosis – very exceptionally in humans
* Chlamydia – causes miscarriages in sheep but probably not in humans
* Various streptococci – miscarriages in horses but unlikely in women
* Mycoplasmas – often blamed for all sorts of disasters with little evidence

Whether any of these bacteria definitely cause human miscarriage is surprisingly uncertain. In any case, this whole argument is not terribly relevant, as a simple course of antibiotics cures all of them very effectively.

Illness   Many illnesses can cause miscarriage. Perhaps the commonest are those which cause a temporary high fever (such as very severe influenza). You are unlikely to get the same illness in two pregnancies, but there are a few conditions that your doctor may want to check you for. These include very high blood pressure (extremely unusual), kidney disease (rare), thyroid problems (less than 1 per cent of miscarriages) and diabetes.

Some viruses cause miscarriage. This is because the foetus can develop abnormally so that a natural abortion happens. The most important is German measles (the medical name is rubella). If you do not have antibodies against this – which can be discovered by a simple blood test – it is wise for you to get immunized before attempting to get pregnant.

Exposure to poisons or toxins   Certain chemicals can lead to miscarriage. These include lead, some insecticides, thalidomide, alcohol, marijuana and nicotine. Although it is most unlikely that any poison with which you have recently come into contact would cause a problem, it is obviously wise to avoid unnecessary exposure to poisonous substances.

Women prone to miscarriage, and pregnant women who have been infertile, should give up smoking – unless they are about to throw themselves under a bus.

Immunological factors There is some evidence that you can miscarry if you and your partner are immunologically compatible. This means if you both have similar tissue types, any foetus you produce may result in a kind of rejection of the foetus by the uterus. Although this is a rare cause of miscarriage, there is some evidence that it may be worth investigating if extensive tests have failed to turn up any other reason for your repeated miscarriages.

Each baby that is born is unique and is different from its parents. One of the remarkable features of pregnancy is the fact that a baby that is quite different from its mother is retained in the uterus without being rejected. In that sense it is quite unlike a transplanted organ such as a kidney. Normally the body rejects foreign tissues, and this rejection phenomenon protects us from harbouring damaged tissue or infection. Curiously, the baby in the uterus is not rejected and the reason for this is not quite clear. Surprisingly, a problem seems to occur if the baby is very similar to its mother and is not immunologically different. For reasons that are not fully understood, miscarriage seems to be more common if there is a high degree of immunological compatibility between mother and baby. This is one of the reasons, for example, why inbreeding of some animals is quite difficult and why abortion occurs more frequently when the foetus is produced as a result of union between close relatives. If you and your partner have similar tissue types, any baby you produce may be rejected and so miscarried. Under these circumstances some doctors believe that it is worth immunizing the mother against her partner's tissues so that any pregnancy is seen by her body to be unique. This kind of treatment is still experimental, and your doctor will need to discuss with you ways in which this problem can be investigated.

Some women who repeatedly miscarry are found to have other

evidence of an immune problem, even though they are entirely fit and well in themselves. In particular, mild affection by the immune disorder disseminated lupus seems to be associated with miscarriage. Other women, who are rather similar, have evidence of an immune problem with their blood vessels. Both these kinds of problem can be evaluated by taking blood tests for the so-called lupus anticoagulant and the anticardiolipin antibody.

PREVENTING MISCARRIAGES

There are a number of ways to reduce the risk of miscarriage, and these are helpful whatever the cause may be.

Rest   The more you relax and take it easy, the better the blood flow to the baby and the more quiet your uterus will be. You should avoid getting up too early and should get to bed at a reasonable time. It is a good idea to take temporary leave from work if you can, at least until the pregnancy is firmly established at about ten weeks or so. If you have repeated miscarriages at a particular time, you should aim to take it really easy at that stage. Don't think of yourself as an invalid though – refusing to leave the house or shop, avoiding any social life at all, may make you more tense and is not likely to help. The aim should be not to get overtired; when you feel tired, make polite excuses and take it easy, with your legs up. Two hours in bed during the afternoon, if you can afford this luxury, is worth considering.

If you have suffered many repeat abortions your doctor may suggest a period of rest in the hospital. Although hospitals are hardly ever relaxing places, hospital bed rest is an option that is worth a try. Why this works we do not know, but the figures show that this is one of the best ways of helping women who have had several miscarriages. At Hammersmith it is our practice to keep women in the hospital until the fourteenth week if they wish, and the excellent results prove the value of this approach.

Diet   A well-balanced diet is important. Small regular meals are advisable and your main need is for fast-acting carbohydrate, such as glucose tablets, high-fibre biscuits or bars, to maintain your energy stores. You certainly do not need a lot of fats, although if you want to eat them, don't feel guilty. You shouldn't worry too much about weight gain at this stage of pregnancy and you should eat what you most enjoy.

Many women feel quite sick in early pregnancy and are not up to eating large quantities of anything. Don't worry about this. Actually, feeling sick is a sign that your pregnancy is thriving and, in my experience, if you feel sick you are less likely to miscarry.

Constipation If you allow yourself to become very constipated indeed, this could encourage a miscarriage. If you have to keep straining very heavily to pass a motion, you might endanger a pregnancy which is already at risk of miscarriage. For this reason, some doctors advise extra fibre in the diet (such as wholemeal bread, fruit and vegetables). They may also suggest a little senna to keep you regular. Don't take laxatives with a vigorous action as these may actually increase the risk. Your doctor will advise you about which laxatives are safe for you.

Iron and folic acid tablets Although people say being short of iron makes miscarriage more likely, this is generally untrue. If you are not anaemic, iron supplements are quite unnecessary until about the twenty-eighth week. Many women don't like taking iron tablets during pregnancy because they can cause an upset stomach. Don't feel that you need to take iron.

Some clinics prescribe a small amount of folic acid. This causes no upset and is the one vitamin that is genuinely valuable if you have a tendency to miscarry, so it is probably wise to take it from the very beginning of pregnancy.

Aspirin, steroids and anticoagulant therapy Women with immune problems such as disseminated lupus or a raised anti-cardiolipin antibody (see page 107) may benefit from daily treatment with aspirin tablets. This is still experimental, but at least harmless. We have treated a number of women with evidence of these disorders with daily aspirin tablets after repeated miscarriages, and they have subsequently delivered healthy children.

Corticosteroids (various forms of cortisone) and anticoagulants (such as heparin) are also under investigation and may prove beneficial. As they are much more risky drugs to give, closer supervision is required than is the case with aspirin. Their use is still experimental, but there is hope that they will be valuable.

Alcohol and smoking   A little alcohol (one or two drinks a week) is not harmful and may even help by relaxing you and quietening the uterus. Smoking has no good effect and may reduce the blood supply to the baby. Unless giving up smoking makes you feel like climbing the kitchen wall, give up – preferably before you get pregnant.

Travel   If you can avoid it, don't go. Short, untiring journeys are fine and gentle train journeys will do no harm. However, it is foolish to go on long flights or skiing holidays in early pregnancy if you are prone to miscarry. Apart from anything else, it puts the doctors you know best out of reach. Moreover, if you do start to bleed, you will find it difficult to forgive yourself even if the trip wasn't the cause of the trouble.

Sex   A difficult one, this! If you have regularly miscarried it is probably sensible to avoid sex in early pregnancy, at least until about the twelfth to the fourteenth week. Sexual activity just may stimulate the uterus and encourage unwanted contractions; certainly some miscarriages seem to be preceded by sexual activity. If you do suddenly feel very amorous and get carried away, don't spend the rest of the week feeling desperately guilty. The chances of miscarriage are very remote and the effect will probably be fairly immediate in any case.

Sport   This is best avoided, as is sun-bathing – lying in the sun for long periods can raise the body temperature, and it is thought that this might harm the foetus. A little gentle swimming will do no harm, but avoid tennis or more strenuous sport. It is obviously unwise to provoke your body deliberately into rejecting the baby.

A woman of thirty-two came to see me in early pregnancy. She was in good health and had never been pregnant before. My examination revealed a normal eight-week pregnancy. There was something about her attitude that slightly troubled me, although I couldn't quite put my finger on it. At the end of the consultation she asked if there were any activities she should avoid that might damage the pregnancy. Knowing that a normal pregnancy in a woman not prone to abort can hardly ever be damaged even by vigorous sport, I remarked she should feel free to do whatever she pleased but somewhat jokingly said that riding a horse was rather unwise.

She returned four weeks later for an antenatal appointment complaining: 'What an awful gynaecologist you are. I've been riding to hounds three times a week for the last month but try as I might I can't get rid of this pregnancy!'

One moral of this story is that you should never feel too bad about what you do in early pregnancy. If you are lucky enough to have achieved a normal implantation, your chances of a baby are really quite high.

Many women blame themselves for miscarrying. They feel that if only they had done less, rested more or altered their lives in some way, the loss could have been avoided. This is wrong; although I have suggested various ways to help yourself, it cannot be denied that the effect of all these measures is marginal at best. The truth is that it is very hard to damage a completely normal pregnancy, no matter what you do. If you miscarry for any of the more specific reasons described earlier in this chapter, special treatment will be needed.

Genetic causes   Tests can be done on the aborted embryo to see if the chromosomes are normal. Parents can also be screened by blood tests. If your blood tests are abnormal, you can get advice from your clinic about the likelihood of your having repeated miscarriages.

Hormonal problems   If you have hormonal imbalance, it too can be detected before pregnancy by blood tests, and corrected with hormone pills. Clomiphene or steroids are the drugs most commonly given; with them you have a 90 per cent chance of getting a pregnancy to stay put eventually, if your problem is hormonal.

If insufficient progesterone seems to be your problem, your doctor will advise you. He or she may give you progesterone after ovulation, either as an injection or pessaries, which you put into the vagina at night (this treatment may also be given to some women who don't ovulate properly or who are having test-tube baby treatment – see Chapters 3 and 10). The treatment is controversial because many experts do not think that 'replacement' therapy of this sort is either effective or necessary. We sometimes give it at Hammersmith, but we are not entirely convinced of its effectiveness.

GnRH treatment   GnRH analogues are now widely used in test-tube baby treatment to suppress the pituitary before starting HMG injections (page 48). I mentioned earlier that some women who have abnormally high levels of LH are sometimes prone to miscarriage. In such cases, treatment with a GnRH analogue, such as Buserelin, to suppress these levels, followed by injections of gonadotrophin (Pergonal or Humegon) to induce normal ovulation, may be recommended. The treatment is still rather experimental and needs careful monitoring with ultrasound and blood hormone tests. However, there is increasing evidence that it may be helpful if this is really your problem.

Uterine abnormalities can easily be detected by x-rays (hysterosalpingography) and then treated surgically (see Chapter 5).

Cervical trouble (cervical incompetence)   This can be treated by your cervix being repaired before you get pregnant, or being stitched shut once you are. Most doctors much prefer to stitch the cervix shut when a woman is pregnant. Although this may seem like shutting the stable door a bit too late, it is the safer and more effective treatment. These stitches are put in around fourteen weeks, before cervical incompetence can cause miscarriage. The stitch must be removed before you deliver. This does not require anaesthesia, but of course it does mean that you will need a new stitch put in with each pregnancy (see page 91).

Illnesses such as high blood pressure, kidney disease, thyroid problems and diabetes your doctor will already know about from your medical history, and special precautions will be taken during pregnancy to keep these under control.

COPING WITH A MISCARRIAGE

Having a miscarriage at any time is a shock. It is really a loss of life within you as well as an event which makes you unwell and depressed. This is much worse if you have had difficulty getting pregnant or if you have already had a miscarriage. Doctors and friends feel helpless and are only able to offer platitudes. Inevitably, doctors are trained to heal people. They find it very difficult to deal with this condition, which occurs so often in spite of treatment, after weeks of rest, and when it is so frequently inexplicable. This makes mere words sound pointless. It may seem to you, if this has been a recent problem of yours, that what is written here is empty.

To make matters worse, the event itself can be very unhappy. Apart from childbirth, miscarriage is almost the commonest reason for a younger woman to enter hospital. Unfortunately, for this very reason hospital staff tend to treat a miscarriage as routine, and do not always seem as helpful and reassuring as they might be. Because the vast majority of women who miscarry go on to have a perfectly normal pregnancy within a few months, the staff sometimes appear a little unaware of your distress.

I think it is important to recognize that a miscarriage is a loss of life and not something that can be brushed away. You have been bereaved and it is important to cry, to mourn. This in itself is the most important part of the healing process. You will naturally feel doubly anxious and nervy during a future pregnancy, but there are some very positive aspects. The figures clearly show that even women who miscarry many, many times are likely to conceive normally eventually. You have at some time to ask yourself how far you are prepared to try, how much trauma you are able to take. I have seen several women with a normal delivery after ten or twelve miscarriages. Of course, if you do persist and succeed eventually, this will not wipe out your earlier distress, but it will not have been in vain.

If you have been infertile as a result of tubal disease or a hormonal problem, a miscarriage is proof that you can get pregnant. You should see this as a sign of real hope that you can conceive. We have analysed the figures for women who miscarry after tubal surgery or in vitro fertilization. It is clear that, providing treatment is continued, the chances of a successful pregnancy are

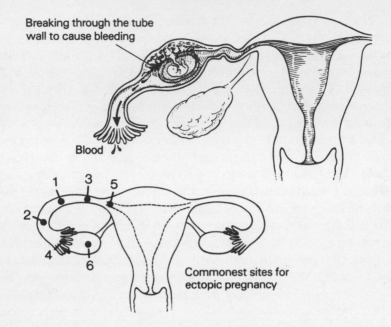

Breaking through the tube
wall to cause bleeding

Blood

1 3 5

2

4

6

Commonest sites for
ectopic pregnancy

much better than even. Remember that a miscarriage is sure
evidence that your tubes are open, that you do ovulate and that the
sperm are fertile.

ECTOPIC PREGNANCY

An ectopic pregnancy takes place when an embryo grows outside
the uterine cavity. What actually happens is that after fertilization
the egg does not manage to travel as far as the uterus, but stops on
its way where it sticks and grows. The usual place is the fallopian
tube (about 96 per cent), but occasionally implantation happens in
other places – either the ovary, abdominal cavity outside the uterus,
or the wall of the uterus where the tube enters the uterine cavity.
There is either not enough room for a pregnancy to grow properly
or the afterbirth (placenta) cannot form normally so ectopic
pregnancies die, or they start to bleed vigorously. If the pregnancy
dies, it is very similar to a miscarriage, except that this ectopic
miscarriage continues inside you and the bleeding cannot escape.

The bleeding is caused by the placenta outgrowing the tissues around it. It can be so heavy that it becomes life threatening.

Ectopic pregnancies are quite common – in the UK about one in two hundred and fifty pregnancies implant outside the uterus, and they are more likely with certain types of infertility (see below). Although having an ectopic is extremely depressing – even worse than having a miscarriage because of the pain and shock – it is worth remembering that women who have ectopics have demon-strated an ability to get pregnant. Like a miscarriage, this shows that they are ovulating, that the sperm is fertile and the eggs are capable of forming embryos. We find it most worthwhile to treat people for infertility who have previously had ectopics, as often the outlook for a successful pregnancy in the end is much better than it is for many infertile women. One treatment is unquestionably in vitro fertilization and we find that it has produced excellent results.

WHAT CAUSES AN ECTOPIC PREGNANCY?

This is not fully understood. But there are several conditions that make it more likely:

1. If the tube has already been damaged, or is partly blocked and the ectopic pregnancy implants in a scarred part of the tube
2. After test-tube baby treatment, probably because the embryo leaves the uterus spontaneously after it is transferred (see Chapter 10)
3. Some women who wear a coil are prone to ectopic pregnancy
4. If you have already had one ectopic pregnancy another one is rather more likely because one of the tubes is damaged.

What are the symptoms?

Usually there is quite a lot of pain, often to one side of the abdomen, together with light bleeding from the vagina. Most women feel pregnant and normally a pregnancy test will be positive, unless the ectopic has already started to die. Then there may be internal bleeding and this makes you feel unwell.

All these symptoms are likely to start very early in pregnancy and you may not have even missed your period. Ectopic pregnancy is rare after about the tenth week, so if you get these symptoms later in pregnancy they probably mean an ordinary miscarriage. If you have any of these symptoms, it is vital that you contact your doctor.

Treatment

The first thing is for a diagnosis to be made. Your doctor will want to do a special test for pregnancy (probably a blood test to detect very small amounts of the pregnancy hormone – see Chapter 3). If there is any doubt about the diagnosis a laparoscopy will be advised.

Because it is so unsafe to have an ectopic pregnancy inside you, and in any case the foetus can virtually never grow to a viable size, an operation is usually needed to remove it. This is rather like having your appendix removed and is not dangerous, but it means perhaps a week in hospital to recover fully afterwards.

You may wonder whether an ectopic pregnancy can be taken out of the tube and immediately replaced in the uterus. Unfortunately this is not possible at the present time. The problem is that although the embryo may be normal, its blood supply would not regrow if this were done.

One of the difficulties about the surgery is that the ectopic pregnancy may have damaged the tube very considerably, even if it was previously normal. This means that most surgeons prefer to remove both the ectopic and the tube it is in. This means you cannot have another ectopic on this side. It also means you have only one tube to get pregnant with in future. Therefore, some surgeons try to remove the ectopic alone and preserve the tube. This 'conservative' surgery is done increasingly frequently nowadays if the woman is already infertile or if there is trouble with the other tube. Although preserving the tube somewhat increases the possibility of another ectopic, it does give a better chance of normal pregnancy as well. Modern methods of preserving the tube do not seem to increase the risk of another ectopic too much.

Removal of an ectopic pregnancy usually requires an open operation which leaves a cut in the abdomen – rather similar to that used for tubal microsurgery (see page 64). The surgery is simpler than that used for most tubal surgery and is not dangerous. However, because ectopic pregnancies sometimes tend to bleed quite vigorously, your doctor may give you a blood transfusion.

Recently there has been a vogue for removing ectopic pregnancies without opening the abdomen – merely by sucking the pregnancy out of the affected tube during a laparoscopic examination. A few surgeons use this approach in Britain, and this technique is most suitable if the pregnancy is quite early (and therefore small). Your doctor will advise this approach only if he or she has the special expertise and instruments required and if the conditions needed to avoid open surgery are present. Moreover, laparoscopic removal of ectopic pregnancy usually implies that no part of the damaged fallopian tube (containing the ectopic) is removed.

Another recent development, which also reduces the disturbance caused by having an ectopic, is to inject a drug into the ectopic pregnancy which will prevent it from growing. The drug commonly used is called methotrexate and is injected at laparoscopy, or using an ultrasound machine to guide the surgeon. Once the injection is accomplished, the ectopic will frequently slowly be absorbed. This treatment is still rather experimental, but seems to work well in cases where the pregnancy has been caught really early.

What are your chances of having a second ectopic pregnancy? Unfortunately they are increased. If you have already had an ectopic pregnancy, you are about ten times more likely than other women to get another. Nevertheless, the odds are about 25 to 1 against, so you are still far more likely to have a normal pregnancy than to have a second ectopic.

Sometimes women find they are unable to conceive again after an ectopic pregnancy. If this is your problem, the best thing is to get a laparoscopy done to check on the state of your tubes, ovaries and uterus. Having an ectopic often results in some adhesions forming, and these can be seen with a laparoscope. It is usually a simple matter to check on this, and you may even have the problem sorted out at the same time, with the adhesions being divided during laparoscopy. Alternatively, it may be possible to repair the other tube with only a tiny risk of another ectopic. A third possibility will of course be the test-tube baby treatment, which I describe in Chapter 10 and which has a comparatively high success rate after ectopic pregnancy.

8

Reversal of sterilization

Some people who have been sterilized bitterly regret their inability to have any more children afterwards. This chapter is written for these men and women.

WHAT IS STERILIZATION?

Women may be sterilized by tubal ligation, which involves the fallopian tubes being cut and then tied. This operation is usually done through a small cut in the abdomen. It blocks the tubes and prevents the sperm and egg from meeting each other. Alternatively, the tubes can be blocked by a small plastic clip or ring being placed tightly across them. This can be done during a laparoscopy, which avoids the need for a more major operation. Occasionally sterilization is done by removing the tubes completely (salpingectomy); in rare cases it involves removing the uterus (hysterectomy). Except when the uterus has been removed, it may be possible to get treatment to allow you to have another baby.

Men are sterilized by the vas (the tube that carries the sperm) being cut and a stitch tied round it. This little operation, called vasectomy, can normally be done under local anaesthesia. It has been reversed successfully in many cases, where there has not been too much surrounding damage.

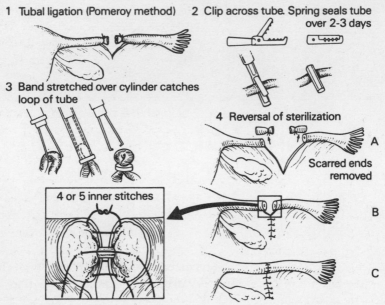

1 Tubal ligation (Pomeroy method)

2 Clip across tube. Spring seals tube over 2-3 days

3 Band stretched over cylinder catches loop of tube

4 Reversal of sterilization

A

Scarred ends removed

4 or 5 inner stitches

B

C

ABOVE, *female sterilization and methods of reversal;* BELOW, *male sterilization – reversal is by rejoining of the vas*

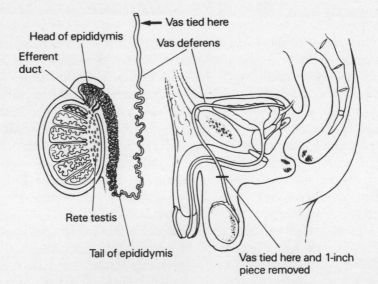

Vas tied here

Head of epididymis

Efferent duct

Vas deferens

Rete testis

Tail of epididymis

Vas tied here and 1-inch piece removed

WHY REVERSAL?

The vast majority of people, about 98 per cent, are very happy with sterilization. Nevertheless, there a few people who are very distressed afterwards, and would do almost anything to get things repaired. One reason why people often regret sterilization is because they have remarried and they want to have a child together. Occasionally people regret sterilization because they find their sexual feelings have altered. Although their problems with sex start after sterilization, it isn't the operation itself that is responsible but rather the knowledge that they can't have a child. If you are in this position, you will recognize these feelings and the feelings of guilt that sometimes go together. They can be so bad that a sterilized woman doesn't feel she's a proper woman any more. Sometimes women are sterilized because of serious illness. Later a new treatment for the illness may mean that the condition can be cured. Because a woman has been sterilized she feels very badly. To my mind, even though sterilization is a voluntary decision, all these cases of infertility deserve sympathy and treatment.

If you happen to be reading this chapter and you are thinking about getting sterilized – a word of warning. It is most unwise to do this if your marriage is breaking up. Sometimes people are fooled into believing that sterilization may save their marriage. In my experience it doesn't. Another bad time to get yourself sterilized is immediately after you have had a pregnancy. Your emotions may not be ready to cope with the thought of another child at that time, but it is probably too early to take a proper decision. Do not get sterilized, either, if you have just been in the unfortunate position of having an abortion. Statistics show you are likely to regret the decision.

What can be done?

If you were sterilized by tubal ligation and you have a reasonable amount of tube remaining, even if only on one side, then an operation may be possible to rejoin the tubes. On the whole, the more tube that has been left undamaged, the better your chances. First you will need to see a sympathetic doctor. More and more family doctors are aware of people having unhappy feelings about sterilization, so this need not be too daunting. The doctor may suggest you talk to the surgeon who originally did your sterilization. If this does not seem appropriate, you will probably be advised to go to a centre that specializes in this kind of operation. If the surgeon feels that it is possible, he will need to do a laparoscopy so that the exact state of your tubes can be assessed. If you have enough tube, you can have an operation to rejoin the tubes. This will require about a week in hospital and the procedure is similar to other types of tubal surgery (see Chapter 4). Within about two weeks, you should be feeling fit enough to have sexual intercourse and it is often possible to conceive immediately.

If you unfortunately have had both tubes completely removed or if the tubes are very badly damaged, your only chance will be the test-tube baby procedure (see Chapter 10). This is usually possible if the scarring has left the ovaries relatively free of adhesions.

What are the chances of success?

As long as the reversal is carried out by someone who specializes in this kind of operation, your chances of getting pregnant are good. The results of surgery are always better if a microscope is used, so you should ask to have the operation done at a unit using microsurgery.

If you have had a clip or ring sterilization and are under the age of thirty-eight, the chance of another baby will be as high as 90 per cent. If your tubes have been cut and tied, the results are not quite as good – about a 75 per cent chance, providing there is not too much damage. Even when there is a lot of damage, more than 50 per cent of women will conceive after microsurgery. If the tubes cannot be operated on because of scarring, the test-tube baby treatment will give you about a 20 per cent chance of conception.

Although there is always a risk of an ectopic pregnancy after any type of tubal surgery, the risk after reversal surgery is actually quite small – about 4 per cent – when microsurgery is used. Most people feel quite happy about accepting such a risk if there is a much better chance of a baby afterwards.

Reversal of male sterilization

Technically, this is not dissimilar to reversal of female sterilization. It involves the vas being rejoined, preferably using microsurgical techniques. Because the vas is a relatively superficial structure in the groin, this operation is not accompanied by much pain, and usually requires only a two or three day stay in hospital.

The success rate varies from centre to centre, but overall about 60 per cent of men who have this operation regain fertility. It is less likely to be successful if you have been sterilized for a long period (say, six years or more) because longstanding blockage of the vas tends to diminish the number of healthy sperm that the testis manufactures. However, vasectomy has no other undesirable effects and in spite of the popular myth, it does not cause loss of virility.

9

Male infertility

The traditional stigma attached to male infertility means quite a lot of men are reluctant to be investigated. Female infertility often causes physical symptoms, so that a woman will go to her doctor with some idea that her body isn't working normally. Male infertility seldom causes symptoms and this is one reason why some men resist becoming involved with tests. This can cause friction between you, especially if there is a likelihood of there being a male problem. Another difficulty is the popular confusion between potency and infertility. A man may feel that if failure to have a baby is his fault, he is not a 'proper' man.

One man who came to our clinic used to have a very active sex life with his wife and they made love three times most nights without fail, to their intense pleasure. When his sperm count was found to be low and the cause of the infertility, their sex life became almost non-existent and he found it difficult even to get an erection. It took a good deal of counselling to overcome the severe blow to his sexual self-esteem, but once the problem had been aired fully, sex became a pleasure again.

It is quite common for people to think that they are inadequate sexually, simply because they can't have children. Men feel this particularly. There is widespread confusion between sexual performance, virility, masculinity and infertility. In fact, there is no connection, and a man's potency is in no way related to his ability to produce sperms. It is equally true that men who are impotent and unable to give their wives any pleasure at all are as likely as the rest of the population to be perfectly fertile.

I know of men who have been so distressed at being infertile that they have committed suicide. Finding their sperm count is low means for some men that they are the responsible party – the guilty one. They have to live with a sense of loss and can, quite illogically, feel deeply ashamed. Frequently the sense of failure spills over into other aspects of a man's life, such as failed professional ambitions. On the woman's side, she may feel angry at being denied a child through no fault of her own. This anger conflicts with her love and feeling for her partner so that she becomes very mixed up. Some women would prefer the problem to be theirs because they feel it would be easier to deal with emotionally. They fear the effect that the diagnosis of male subfertility will have on their partners, and try to protect them by sheltering them from being tested. Others go through all sorts of tests without even telling their husbands that they are attending an infertility clinic. And others find that their partners will not see a doctor at all, nor will they produce sperm for testing. They neither want to go through the ordeal of the test nor admit to what they feel is a reflection on their sexuality. Needless to say, two people are involved when infertility is the problem and you have to find a way of airing the difficulties. It may be very worthwhile having a frank and open discussion with your doctor so that he or she can suggest ways that you can both come to grips with the situation.

Male problems are the reason for about 30 per cent of all infertility. In the past, male infertility was regarded as a terrible blow as, except in rare cases, it was untreatable. We now understand the causes better and are able to test for them. Consequently there is more hope that something can be done if you have this problem.

WHAT ARE THE CAUSES?

No sperm in the semen

Sometimes no sperm can be found in the seminal fluid. This may be because none are being made by the testicle, or because they are not being ejaculated during orgasm. Failure to ejaculate sperm in spite of their production by the testicle is either because the tubes from the testes to the seminal vesicles are blocked (see the diagram on page 4), or because the muscles that pump semen through the penis are not working properly.

Failure of the testis to produce any sperm at all is, fortunately, pretty rare, with less than 5 per cent of infertile men having this problem. Although ovarian failure in women is frequently treatable with hormones, testicular failure is very difficult to alter. The cause is frequently unknown but occasionally may be due to a hard blow to the testis, such as a sporting injury, a previous severe mumps infection, or damage to the blood supply to the testicle – this is usually due to serious twisting of the testis. If this is the case, the doctor may make the diagnosis easily from discussing your past medical history.

Other reasons for testicular failure are hormonal. Either the pituitary gland is not producing enough hormones to stimulate the testes or the testes are not responding to these hormones. There are various reasons why the testes may not respond to pituitary hormones:

- rare defects from birth (chromosomal)
- undescended and therefore poorly developed testes
- the cells of the testis cannot respond to testosterone (male hormone).

If treatment is possible at all, hormones will be needed (see below).

If the tubes from the testis to the seminal vesicles are blocked the testes may produce sperm but they cannot get into the semen. Blockage of these tubes is a result of scarring, sometimes due to infection such as gonorrhoea or tuberculosis, or occasionally because of injury. You may also have been born with blockages of part of the system of tubes.

Occasionally (in less than 1 per cent of men), the genital muscles do not pump in a properly coordinated way during orgasm. Sperm may enter the bladder and mix with the urine, rather than get into the vagina. This is called retrograde ejaculation and may follow an operation such as removal of the prostate gland. It may also happen if the nerves to the muscles are damaged. Some drugs, particularly tranquillizers, or drugs to control high blood pressure, may also temporarily cause this.

The semen contains few sperm or sperm of poor quality

Over 90 per cent of male problems are due to this. There are very many reasons why your sperm count may be low, but most often the real cause cannot be discovered.

Hormonal problems may drastically reduce sperm quality. Any that prevent all sperm production (as I described above) can just result in fewer normal sperm being produced. The more severe the hormonal problem, the worse will be the sperm quality.

Abnormal blood vessels around the testicle may be associated with poor sperm quality. You may have enlarged veins draining the testicles, rather like varicose veins. This condition is known as varicocoele, and is thought by some people to cause overheating of the testis: the blood in the enlarged veins may keep the testis at a higher temperature than normal. The reason why varicocoele causes some men to be infertile but not others is not yet known. Overheating has not been proved to be the cause.

An infection that has lasted a long time is sometimes thought to cause poor sperm quality. An infection of the prostate gland may be found in a few men with poor sperm. Some doctors believe that one group of germs, the mycoplasmas, are particularly likely to cause problems, perhaps by reducing sperm motility.

The mycoplasmas are one of the germs that have recently come under considerable scientific scrutiny. There is good evidence in animals that these organisms may interfere with the ability of sperm to fertilize an egg. Although the germs are not at all dangerous in themselves and hardly ever cause health-threatening infections, antibiotics may be prescribed if they are thought to be affecting your sperm quality.

Environmental reasons

Very frequently there are simple environmental reasons. Among these are severe pressure of work, smoking and excessive alcohol. Some drugs can also depress your sperm count, and acute illness or fever may reduce sperm numbers. This is encouraging, as the problem can fairly easily be put right. Among the most common factors affecting sperm count are:

Being overweight   Although many obese men are fertile, there is an increased chance of infertility if you are overweight.

Smoking can affect sperm counts. It may have no effect on many men with completely normal or high sperm counts, but if you are prone to underproduce sperm, you may have a catastrophic drop in sperm numbers and quality if you smoke.

Alcohol   Like tobacco, alcohol is a poison that damages your cells. Excessive drinking is likely to reduce your ability to make sperm. Different people have a different tolerance, but on page 138 I give some idea of the average amount it would be sensible to drink if your sperm count is low.

Drugs   There are many drugs that reduce sperm count. On the list of 'social' drugs is marijuana. There is no doubt that marijuana can have a powerful effect on some men and its use should be avoided if you are infertile. Medicinal drugs that are sometimes thought to depress sperm count include:

- Antidepressants
- Antimalarial drugs
- Antihypertensives (for treating high blood pressure)
- Sulphasalazine (used for colitis)
- Cytotoxic drugs (for blood disorders and certain malignancies)
- Furadantin (used for bladder infections)

- Corticosteroids (this is not proved but they may affect some men).

Excessive exercise Regular sport, jogging or cycling promotes well-being, but there is evidence that excessive strenuous exercise may affect sperm production. We know that some athletes at the peak of training have reduced sperm counts that return to normal when they exercise less and gain a little weight.

Your job and the stresses of daily life This is a most difficult factor to weigh up. It is always a problem to understand just which aspects of anyone's life may be contributing to poor fertility. At particular risk are people such as the high-powered executive, who is constantly flying around the world and is under pressure all the time. To make matters worse, he may often be away from home for long periods, perhaps at those times when his wife is most fertile. Apart from reducing the chance of conception, time away from home throws added strain on the sexual and marital relationship, compounding stress. These professional pressures are often worst in your thirties and early forties, when you are carving out a career. Yet this may be the best time for you to have a child. If you leave things too late, your partner will be less fertile.

Other occupations associated with sperm problems include long-distance driving or jobs where you are exposed to poisonous substances such as lead; for example, lead fumes in a bus depot. Men exposed to excessive vibration such as boiler makers or pneumatic drill operators, or in any other jobs where the environment is very tiring or stressful, may also be affected.

If you have intercourse too frequently Some people think the quality and quantity of their sperm may be reduced. This is not proved. We know that many men who have intercourse several times a day are completely fertile.

The sperm are abnormal

Sometimes sperm that look normal under the microscope are actually chemically abnormal. Although these may be produced in large numbers, they may be incapable of fertilizing an egg. It is unusual to find the reason for the abnormality. Sometimes, though, it is due to a simple bacterial infection, treatable with antibiotics.

Immunological problems

This is the reason for about 5 to 10 per cent of male infertility. For reasons that are not yet known, some men form antibodies to their own sperm. The sperms are 'sensed' to be 'foreign' and are attacked by the body just as the body attacks other foreign proteins or bacteria and cells. Sperm antibodies may prevent the sperm from being released at all.

Intercourse

Difficulty with sexual intercourse is very rarely the cause of infertility (less than 1 per cent of male infertility). Sexual difficulties can result in sperm not being ejaculated into the vagina. The commonest problem is what is called premature ejaculation, when the man has his orgasm before he is able to get the penis deep into the vagina. This is more likely in very young men and can be overcome with patience and practice.

There are many other reasons for difficulty with intercourse, and these are outside the scope of this book. Sexual problems need specialized help and the best people to consult are often counsellors trained in marriage guidance. Your doctor should suggest the best sources of help available to you. Though you may feel embarrassed to discuss this, you will find you get sympathetic advice from the people familiar with these problems.

Anatomical abnormality

This is also very rare. The commonest of these rare problems is the condition known as hypospadias, when the urethra, the tube running through the penis, opens into the outside world underneath the penis or even near the scrotum (see the diagram on page 4) As with retrograde ejaculation, sperm are not ejaculated into the vagina. This can be treated with a simple operation.

Absence of the vas, or poorly developed testes are other rare anatomical abnormalities (see below).

HOW CAN A PROBLEM WITH THE MAN BE TESTED?

Physical examination

Your doctor will examine you to see whether your testes are descended properly into the scrotum and if they are normal in size. Abnormally small or very soft testes may mean that there is a failure of sperm production. Examination will also be helpful in excluding an anatomical abnormality such as hypospadias or absence of the vas, the main duct which conveys the sperm to the seminal vesicle. Enlargement of the veins around the testicle (varicocoele) can usually be felt during physical examination by a doctor, especially when you stand upright and strain down or cough. Signs of infection may also be picked up.

Semen analysis

This is the most important of all your tests, but it is less unpleasant than it sounds. Semen can be collected during interrupted intercourse or after masturbation. A good infertility clinic will give you clear written instructions about the method of collection they prefer and how quickly you must take it in for analysis. They should also tell you how long before testing you should avoid sex. Some clinics prefer you not to have had intercourse for three days before a test, though opinions vary about how important this is.

Examination of the semen under a microscope will show whether it is normal. The number of sperm is counted, and how well they move around is assessed. The proportion of normal sperm can be estimated. A normal man will usually ejaculate about 1.5 to 6 millilitres of fluid. In a normal test, each millilitre should contain at least twenty million sperm and 60 per cent of these should be normal in shape and size. Good, motile sperm should be capable of swimming vigorously in a straight line.

Chemical tests can also be done on the fluid in which the sperm are ejaculated. The total volume of the ejaculate is also measured, as a very small or very large volume may predispose to infertility. Immediately after ejaculation the semen contains jelly-like particles, but after about thirty minutes these should liquefy more or less completely.

When you return to your doctor to get the result of the sperm count it is well worth making sure that both of you go together. It can be a considerable burden for the woman to go on her own and find out that her man has a problem. Most women do not want to be the one who has to break the news of a low sperm count, because they feel that bad news will be an unexpected hurt. You must remember that perfectly fertile men may from time to time have an abnormal semen test. A single poor test carries no significance, so do not be depressed if the first count is below average.

Findings on semen analysis

1. *Only a few normal sperm are found*: this is a common finding. Some completely normal, fertile men produce only a few normal sperm on a single, isolated occasion. If several tests contain less than twenty million sperm per millilitre this is likely to be a factor causing infertility. A low sperm count can be due to any of the causes described on pages 127–9.

2. *Sperm are present in the semen but few are moving normally*: this is also very common. When there are only a few normally moving sperm the outlook is not as good as it is when there are few sperm showing normal movement. It is usually abnormal to have fewer than 40 per cent of the sperm swimming in a reasonably straight line. The causes include:

- Infection in the semen
- Failure of the testis to produce normal sperm
- Failure of the epididymis to provide the right environment for sperm
- The semen was collected wrongly or was left to stand for too long before being tested
- A varicocoele is present (though it is doubtful that this really is a genuine cause).

3. *If the volume of the ejaculate is below 0.5 millilitres*, this may be due to severe inflammation of the glands that produce seminal fluid or because the tubes conducting the sperm are abnormal (see page 130). However, many normal men produce

a low volume of semen, so this does not necessarily mean that there is something wrong.

4. *No sperm are seen*   This means that the testis is not producing sperm or there is a block in the tubes from the testicle. Very rarely retrograde ejaculation, when semen is ejaculated into the bladder (see above), may be the cause.

5. *A large proportion of the sperm look abnormal*   Again, there are many reasons for the production of abnormal sperms. If the majority of the sperm have minute abnormalities, visible under the microscope, the chance of successful treatment is small. The reasons for abnormal sperm tend to be similar to the reasons in groups 2 and 4 above.

6. *The semen does not liquefy properly*   This unusual problem is usually due to infection or a chemical insufficiency.

7. *The sperm seem stuck to each other or form clumps*   This suggests some infection in the semen or possibly that you have sperm antibodies.

The post-coital test (PCT)

This is described more fully in Chapter 6. A small sample of mucus is sucked from the cervix, usually about six to twenty-four hours after intercourse. It is then examined under a microscope to see if moving sperm are present. Although this test is mostly used to see if there is a problem with your partner's mucus, it can help in assessing the man. If sperm are present, it means that there is no problem with intercourse. If many sperm are moving, even if sperm counts have been low, it suggests that your sperm may be of quite good quality and are capable of fertilization.

Special sperm counts: swim up and velocity testing

We know definitely that, even when the sperm are abnormal, routine sperm counts do not always detect this. Recently, two types of test have been developed which are an improvement on routine analysis. They depend on testing the ability of the sperm to swim. If they swim poorly or slowly, it is possible there may be an abnormality that prevents fertilization. Unfortunately, these abnormalities, which are probably chemical in nature, cannot yet be treated, but knowledge of their existence is an important first step.

The swim up or swim test　　This test involves placing the sperm in a tube with a layer of specially prepared fluid medium on top. Normal sperm should swim into the medium, leaving the abnormal sperm behind at the bottom of the tube. This test is actually used as a method to prepare sperm before using them for in vitro fertilization (see page 152) or some types of artificial insemination, but it can also be used to get an idea of the percentage of normal sperm a man produces. In most laboratories a good swim test should provide at least 500,000 really active sperm from the semen.

Sperm velocity testing　　In this test, sperm are placed in medium under a microscope and repeatedly photographed at intervals of a few seconds. This time-lapse photography can then be analysed and the distance the various sperm have travelled gives a clue to their motility and therefore their health. The most sophisticated velocity testing involves the use of a computer to assess the percentage of sperm that are capable of moving rapidly. The higher the percentage, the better the outlook for fertility.

Hormone tests

These will be suggested only if your sperm count is low. There are three types:

Measurement of the male hormone, testosterone　　This is done by taking a blood sample. If your testosterone level is lower than normal the cells in the testis are probably not working properly. If high, there is the very rare possibility that some of the cells in the testis cannot respond normally to the male hormone. This condition is the cause of less than 1 per cent of male problems but is not usually treatable.

Measurement of the pituitary hormones, LH (luteinizing hormone) and FSH (follicle stimulating hormone)　　These are the same as in the woman (see Chapter 3). If your levels are raised, it means unfortunately that the testicle is not making sperm and generally will not respond to treatment. If your levels are low, the pituitary gland may not be producing enough hormone and there is a possibility at least of hormone treatment being effective.

Measurement of prolactin This is the hormone that in women stimulates milk production from the breast. It is produced by the pituitary gland in men too and can be abnormally high, though this is unusual.

High levels may occasionally be caused by a benign tumour of the pituitary which is easily treatable by minor surgery. The evidence that prolactin really affects sperm production is extremely poor.

Surgical exploration of the testicle

If the other tests have shown no cause, it is possible that your doctor will recommend a minor exploratory operation on one testicle. This is usually done within one day at the hospital, under light general anaesthetic. Your doctor may decide to remove a tiny piece of the testis for examination under the microscope. This will help discover whether the testis is actually manufacturing sperm. It is usual to examine the tube close to the testis, the epididymis, at the same time to see if it looks diseased or blocked.

Your surgeon may also perform a vasogram, which involves injecting a little dye into the vas deferens and then taking an x-ray. This will help pinpoint the exact position of any block in the tubing.

The hamster egg test

We know that some sperm just cannot fertilize an egg. One test, recently devised, involves the use of golden hamster eggs. Specially prepared sperm are taken from the semen and mixed with a number of hamster eggs. In order to make the hamster eggs penetrable by human sperm, these eggs are first chemically stripped of their outer coat, the zona. Eggs so treated are then capable of being penetrated by non-hamster sperm; however, they are not capable of proper fertilization or of growing into embryos. This test is therefore ethically acceptable.

A biologist counts the percentage of 'fertilized' eggs and makes an assessment of the quality of the sperm. If no eggs at all are 'fertilized', there may be something wrong with the sperm. However, there is considerable doubt about how reliable this test is. We know that sometimes, even when it is completely negative, fertilization of human eggs is possible.

The human zona penetration test

Sperm can be mixed with dead human eggs, obtained usually from a 'spare' ovary removed during hysterectomy. This test evaluates the ability of sperm to penetrate the outer layer of the egg. Even if the sperm penetrate the outer layer, there is no risk of an embryo being formed as the egg itself is dead. This test is probably more useful than the hamster egg test in evaluating sperm quality, but more research is needed before we can say how reliable it really is. It is still available only in research centres and is unlikely at present to be done in your case.

In vitro fertilization

'Washed' sperm can be mixed with a live egg taken from your partner just before ovulation. This is, in fact, an extension of the test-tube baby process. If an embryo develops, this is, of course, the best proof that the sperm are capable of normal activity. Any embryo that is obtained can be put back into your partner's uterus, where it may develop into a baby. In many ways this is the ultimate test of sperm function; the reason why it is not done more often is because it is very expensive. Unfortunately it is available only at some of the centres where the test-tube baby treatment is done.

TREATMENT

A large question mark exists over virtually all treatments for improving sperm counts. We still do not understand the reasons why some sperm are healthy, others not. There are several extremely complex chemical processes involved, which are unlikely to be influenced much by simple remedies. However, only one sperm is needed to produce a baby so even men with an apparently hopelessly low sperm count may eventually successfully produce a baby. The message is clear. If sperm are being produced at all, however few, there is always the possibility of success.

Having said that simple remedies are unlikely to influence the complex events that contribute to sperm function, we should now look at various measures that have been tried, some of which are undoubtedly of value.

General health

This is important. There is no doubt that many fertile men are prone to poor sperm counts, which may make them at least temporarily infertile. If your sperm count is marginal or low it is really worthwhile obeying certain health rules to maximize the chances of a baby. The solutions to the environmental hazards described on pages 128–9 are relatively simple, compared with other treatments. You should try to persevere with the suggestions recommended here. However, bear in mind that your sperm count may not actually improve much for the first four months or so.

Being overweight   You should try to lose excessive body weight by going on a suitable diet. It is better to reduce gradually, losing around two pounds (one kilo) each week. Do not try crash dieting, which may lose you dramatic amounts but will probably result in a terrific binge at the end of the starvation, when you put the weight back on again.

Smoking   If you smoke more than eight or ten cigarettes a day and you have a poor sperm count, giving up smoking may be the most important line of treatment. Ideally, you should give up completely. If you are a heavy smoker and you decide to give up, do not expect your sperm count to return to normal levels immediately. It takes just over three months for the testis to make sperm and for them to be transported to the vas ready for ejaculation.

A thirty-three-year-old salesman and his wife came to see me after they had failed to have a baby in the eleven years of their marriage. She ovulated rather poorly and had been on drugs for seven years without a pregnancy. His sperm counts were always low, and artificial insemination had been tried many times without success. We measured his count four times in four successive months. The number of sperm per millilitre varied between four million and nine million, and the motility was never more than 30 per cent; usually about 40 per cent of the sperm showed some microscopic abnormality. I advised him to lose twenty pounds (nine kilos) and cut out smoking – at that time he was smoking thirty-five to forty cigarettes a day. He drove a great deal owing to his work, but he didn't feel he could alter this much.

I saw him three months later. He had cut down to four cigarettes a day and had lost over fourteen pounds (six kilos) in weight. He had continued with his normal work, but was now exercising twice weekly – the first time for years. His sperm count on the day of his appointment was fifty-six million per millilitre and 50 per cent of the sperm were moving normally; about 30 per cent still showed some abnormality in shape. His sperm count remained at this level two months later. Five weeks after the second of these counts, his wife had a positive pregnancy test.

Alcohol   With everyone having a different reaction to drink it is impossible to lay down precise guidelines about what your limit should be. You shouldn't drink more than two or three pints (one to five litres) of beer daily, or more than half a bottle of wine. Spirits are thought to be particularly harmful, and you should limit yourself to two or three measures a day.

Drugs   If you are taking any medically prescribed drugs it is important to discuss this with your doctor. Obviously you can't stop drugs that are important to your health, but a change might be helpful or, alternatively, a different dose.

As mentioned earlier, you should give up all 'social' drugs if you've been in the habit of using them.

Excessive exercise   Regular marathon running or daily vigorous games of squash may be unwise. If you think you have taken physical training too far, it would be sensible to ease off a while to see if your sperm count improves.

The stress of daily life   It is always difficult to know how best to structure your life, but perhaps you need to ask yourself whether you should spend more time at home and duck some of the heaviest commitments at work.

If this is not for you to decide – if you have a tedious, repetitive job that is getting you down, or you are unemployed and this is becoming a strain for you and your partner – a discussion with your doctor or a marriage guidance counsellor may help you arrive at a better way of coping with the tensions.

Other environmental factors   Sometimes men are told to take cold baths and wear loose-fitting pants. There is limited logic behind these suggestions. The testicles hang outside the body in the scrotum. This is nature's way of keeping the testes cooler than body temperature. It seems that sperm production is best when the testis is a degree or two lower than 98.4°F (37°C). It may be that close-fitting pants, such as Y-fronts, cause overheating and some doctors recommend men with low sperm counts to wear loose boxer shorts and even bathe the scrotum daily in very cold water. There is really no proof that any of this will help, and some couples feel it adds an element of torture to what is already an unpleasant situation. On the other hand, it does no harm and may be worth a go if only because it means that you are doing everything possible. Wearing loose-fitting pants makes reasonable sense, and it seems a good idea to avoid very hot baths and saunas. I would avoid cold water treatments, however, as I am very unconvinced that they can be of real help. You may be interested to know that in some parts of the world (especially Japan) hot baths have been used as a method of male contraception.

Drug treatments

These are the most controversial. Many drugs have been tried to improve sperm quality and numbers, and that fact itself demonstrates the lack of success. The truth is that, except in a few specific cases, drugs are not likely to make much difference. Although this is depressing news, it is important that you recognize it from the outset, to avoid wasting a lot of time on different but equally ineffective drugs. Those that may be tried are:

Testosterone (male hormone)   Large doses of testosterone actually reduce your sperm count, so there is no point in long-term testosterone treatment. Some men, though, have a 'rebound' effect. A short course of treatment with large doses of testosterone (given usually by injection) temporarily suppresses their sperm production. When the drug is stopped, the testis may 'rebound' and there are claims that as many as 50 per cent of men will have a marked improvement in sperm count, though this effect will last only a short time.

Gonadotrophins (pituitary hormones FSH and LH)   These may be given by injection (Pergonal). Alternatively, LH may be given alone, usually as HCG (human chorionic gonadotrophin or Pregnyl, Profasi). Claims have been made that, because these compounds increase the activity of the testicle, sperm counts may improve. It is usually claimed that sperm numbers rather than motility are improved by these drugs, but in any case their effect seems variable. They have been proved effective only for men with a pituitary abnormality, when normal production of FSH is decreased. These drugs are extremely expensive and treatment is lengthy; my feeling is that they are not justified unless you have a definite and well-defined hormone problem.

Bromocriptine (Parlodel)   Probably the only reason to give this drug to men is when there is a specific pituitary problem. If excessive prolactin is being produced it may just be helpful.

Clomiphene (Clomid) and tamoxifen are mostly used to stimulate the pituitary in women (see Chapter 3); they also affect the ovaries and uterus directly – sometimes unfavourably. They have occasionally been used to raise testosterone production by the testis in the hope of improving the sperm count. Success has been very variable. We have used Clomid and tamoxifen a lot in the past, but have never been convinced that anyone we have given them to has benefited. We have now almost given up using this group of drugs for male infertility.

Mesterolone (Pro-Viron)   This is a synthetic by-product of testosterone and is claimed to improve sperm motility and possibly sperm numbers. It is probably the most widely used drug for male infertility but there is disappointingly little hard evidence that it improves fertility. We have used this drug extensively for very many years on large numbers of men; although some have shown improvements in sperm count, it is quite possible that the sperm count improved by itself. Very few of the men taking mesterolone have produced pregnancies, probably no more than would have done so by chance.

Antibiotics   These are slightly different. There is little doubt that if you have an infection impairing sperm quality, the chance of fertilization is reduced. Taking antibiotics may solve this problem. The treatment is normally for four to six weeks.

Immune therapy   If you have poor sperm counts due to antibodies to your own sperm, drugs may just be helpful. Corticosteroids are most commonly used, either prednisone or ACTH. You may have to take the drugs intermittently for several months, and in quite high doses. These drugs can be effective only if the testis is not irreversibly damaged. The usual practice is to give high doses of prednisone for seven days or so each month to coincide with your partner's fertile period.

Doses of steroids in the large amounts needed to suppress antibodies have certain risks, and you should follow your doctor's advice carefully. You should not continue to take steroids for more than three or four months. It is claimed that about half of all men with antibodies may be helped by these drugs, that is, about 3 or 4 per cent of all infertile men.

Another way of getting around the problem of antibodies is to have your sperm 'washed'. The semen are taken and mixed in specially prepared solutions. The 'washed' sperm can then be inseminated into your partner's cervix with a little syringe. So far this has had only limited success.

If your sperm show persistent evidence of being killed by your own antibodies, artificial insemination with donor sperm may be worth considering (see Chapter 11).

Surgical treatments

Dealing with a varicocoele   Surgical correction of a varicocoele is very simple, but there are conflicting opinions about its value. The problem is that about 20 per cent of both fertile and infertile men have a varicocoele, and this seems no disadvantage to a fertile man. It is thought, though, that there is more chance of infertility if there is abnormal bloodflow in these varicose veins (see page 127).

The operation, called ligation, is either to tie off the abnormal vessels or to block them, usually with a chemical injection. If the injection method is used, a local anaesthetic is generally all that is needed. X-rays may be taken to confirm that the veins are effectively blocked. Some surgeons claim that at least 70 per cent of men will show an improvement in sperm count within three months of this treatment. Others are less optimistic and some have not found that ligation of a varicocoele produces any improvement.

Varicocoeles are painless and whether treated or not they do not interfere with sex.

Unblocking the tubing (see the diagram on page 4)   These tubes are very tiny; the epididymis has an inner diameter of less than 0.2 millimetres, that is, the thickness of a piece of very fine cotton thread. The vas is much thicker externally but it too is very narrow internally. If the blocked portion has to be removed and the tubing rejoined, the best results are obtained by microsurgery, with stitches so fine that they can hardly be seen at all with the naked eye. Although the surgery is technically difficult and you will need a general anaesthetic, recovery is very quick and there is hardly any pain so intercourse is not affected. You need stay in hospital only for a few days.

Results of microsurgery vary, depending on the position and extent of the block. If the tubing has been blocked for a long time, the testis tends gradually to stop producing sperm. Unfortunately, if production stops altogether, more sperm may not be made even when the tubing is unblocked. Eight per cent of infertile men have a block and 20 to 30 per cent will produce normal sperm after this type of operation.

In vitro fertilization and GIFT

There is increasing interest in the use of test-tube baby treatment or in vitro fertilization (IVF) and gamete intra-fallopian transfer (GIFT) treatment (see page 162) for male infertility. Whilst I do not consider GIFT treatment to be particularly helpful, there is no doubt that IVF has made a huge impact on the treatment of male infertility. For a full account of this, see Chapter 10.

ARTIFICIAL INSEMINATION WITH THE MALE PARTNER'S SEMEN

Insemination with the partner's semen (AIH) may be recommended in some cases when the sperm count is poor. Sperm are inseminated by one of three methods rather than natural intercourse being allowed:

- insemination into the cervix
- insemination into the cervix with your partner's sperm which has been specially processed first
- insemination directly into the uterus itself.

Insemination into the cervix   Semen, usually produced by masturbation, is injected directly into the vagina through a small plastic tube. You need to lie on a couch with your knees up for about five minutes for this; it is without discomfort. This kind of insemination is used for couples having difficulties with sexual intercourse; it may also be useful in the rare event of your having an anatomical problem with the uterus or cervix which prevents sperm finding the right place. Although this is controversial, I feel it usually has very little point if your man has a low count because natural intercourse achieves the same end – that is, introduction of sperms into the cervical canal. One theoretical advantage of AIH is that insemination can be made at the most fertile moment – just before ovulation.

Insemination with your partner's sperm which has been specially processed   The sperm are prepared after being produced by

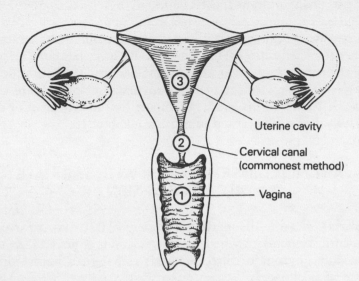

Uterine cavity

Cervical canal
(commonest method)

Vagina

The three points at which sperm may be inseminated

masturbation. They may be 'washed', that is, the semen is repeatedly mixed with special laboratory fluid (medium) and the sperm then removed by centrifugal force, by spinning the tube containing them. Alternatively, the sperm may be subjected to the 'swim up'. The semen is mixed with medium, healthy sperm are allowed to swim up to the surface under their own steam and they are drawn off by suction with a glass tube. These healthy, concentrated sperm may then be inseminated into the cervix.

Either of these methods may be used if there are large numbers of dead sperm in the semen, or many dead cells present. Strictly speaking, no real concentration of semen takes place, just a purification. These methods may also be used if there are sperm antibodies present, as the washing process may get rid of these.

Another method of preparing semen involves using a split ejaculate. Most of the sperm are normally ejected from the penis at the beginning of ejaculation. The rest of the seminal fluid tends to contain inessential constituents, including water. Even subfertile men often produce most of the sperm at the beginning of ejaculation. To collect the best sperm and 'concentrate' them, your doctor may suggest obtaining a split ejaculate. During masturbation, the first half of the fluid is collected in one sterile pot and the second half in another. It is a well-known but little published fact that professional jugglers are best at doing this test. Examination under the microscope can then confirm whether most of the sperm are truly in the first half of the ejaculate. If they are, then only this part of the semen is inseminated. Split ejaculates are useful when the motility of sperm is good, but the total number is low.

When used appropriately, these methods can result in pregnancy in around 30 per cent of subfertile couples.

Intrauterine insemination   Occasionally doctors advise insemination directly into the uterus itself, bypassing the cervix. This is usually done when there is a cervical problem (Chapter 5). However, intrauterine insemination is now being used for some male infertility, especially when the count is poor. A fine tube containing sperm is inserted through the cervix and just into the uterus. This can cause minor discomfort but there should be no pain.

Neat semen, unwashed, cannot be used because of a risk of infection or an allergic reaction. The sperm need to be prepared in the laboratory either by being washed or by the swim up method described above. Although not enough people have yet had this treatment for it to be properly evaluated, early results are somewhat encouraging and a few doctors have had a success with up to 40 per cent of couples.

What are the disadvantages of insemination with your partner's sperm?

The disadvantages are so great that I would advise this treatment for only a limited time, say, no more than six months.
  They include:

1. The process itself tends to be very clinical and unspontaneous, and for some people this is almost worse than being infertile. There is no doubt that this treatment invades your sex life to a greater extent than most doctors are prepared to admit.
2. The man may not be able to masturbate to order. This will at least be embarrassing and at worst cause feelings of guilt,

frustration and anger. A great deal of patience and understanding is needed between partners.

3. Reasonably precise timing of ovulation is necessary. Tem-
    perature charting is insufficient and your clinic will probably
    want you to go in for blood tests, ultrasound or both.

4. Collecting a split ejaculate requires considerable manual dex-
    terity right at the moment of orgasm.

5. Sperm washing or the swim up require advanced laboratory
    facilities, which are available only in relatively few centres as
    the laboratory work is expensive and time-consuming.

6. Insemination is unlikely to work in the first month. To give a
    chance of sperm being present at the right moment, insemina-
    tion may be done two or three times each month, and even so
    most couples who succeed do so only after several months with
    insemination. Here then is a paradox, because perseverance
    may be needed and this becomes more difficult as months go
    by without success. Many couples find AIH so frustrating and
    invasive of their sex lives that they may give up after three or
    four months.

10

IVF Treatment

IN VITRO FERTILIZATION – THE TEST-TUBE BABY TECHNIQUE

The idea behind the so-called test-tube baby treatment is very simple. It involves removing an egg from the woman's ovary, collecting and cleaning her partner's sperm, mixing the sperm and egg in the laboratory and, if fertilization occurs, inserting the developing egg or embryo into the woman's uterus. The embryo is put back into the mother's body about two or three days after fertilization, while it is still a group of cells and long before any organs have developed.

The procedure has various medical names. It is normally referred to as in vitro fertilization; *in vitro* is from the Latin meaning glass, because the egg is fertilized in laboratory glassware. In vitro fertilization is most frequently called IVF for short. It may also be called extra-corporeal fertilization, extra-corporeal meaning outside the body, from the Latin, *corpus* body. You may read or hear, too, of the term embryo transfer, which refers simply to the embryo being put back into the uterus. The term artificial insemination is sometimes confused with IVF, but this is entirely different (and is described in Chapter 9).

IVF treatment requires a great deal of commitment from the couple and from the staff carrying it out. You may be asked to attend clinics at unsociable hours and at repeated intervals. There is no doubt that you will be required to make some sacrifices to have the best chance of success. For example, some women find it difficult to carry on working during a treatment cycle. So it is important that you are certain you want to try everything to get a child of your own, otherwise it really is not worth the effort. If you have any doubts at any stage of your treatment it is essential that you discuss them fully with a member of the team, who will often themselves be making considerable sacrifices to make sure you get the best possible care. If you are doubtful, it is much better to be frank and ask for treatment to be delayed until you are absolutely ready to go through with it all.

FOR WHOM IS IVF SUITABLE?

Most definitely this is not right for everyone who is infertile. Newspapers and television programmes have tended to give the wrong impression that it can be used for most, if not all infertility. Relatively speaking, IVF has a low rate of success everywhere, and this is likely to remain the case in the near future. Success rates on paper, in newspapers, magazines and on television always sound better than they really are because they don't take into account people who are unsuitable or early failures of treatment. It is therefore realistic for it to be tried only when there is no satisfactory alternative or when other treatments have a very remote chance of a success.

Since the process basically simply bypasses the fallopian tubes, you still need to have a more or less normal uterus, for example, and ovaries capable of producing some eggs when stimulated. The main reasons for trying IVF are:

- When surgery to correct tubal disease has been unsuccessful
- When the tubes are so badly damaged that tubal surgery has less chance of success than in vitro fertilization
- When the tubes are both damaged and the husband's sperm count is also on the low side
- For many cases of male infertility, when at least some normal sperm are being produced
- For women who fail to ovulate naturally and have not

responded adequately to HMG treatment. Such patients must be capable of producing some eggs

- When there is a major problem with the cervix which prevents sperm reaching the right place, and other treatments have failed
- For a substantial number of (but by no means all) cases of unexplained infertility or endometriosis, providing they have been fully investigated first

Too many clinics use in vitro fertilization far too soon, or when the reason for the infertility is not clear and there has been a failure to carry out adequate tests. At Hammersmith we believe that it is much more satisfactory to carry out proper tests first, find the cause and treat it accordingly. When this is done, far fewer couples turn out to require IVF.

FOR WHOM IS IVF NOT USUALLY SUITABLE?

Regrettably there are very many women who are really unsuitable for routine IVF. These include:

- Women who have had their uterus removed
- Women with excessive scarring or abnormalities of the uterus which make implantation of an embryo impossible – such as a congenital problem, or large fibroids
- Anyone who has had extensive tuberculosis of the uterus, leaving a great deal of heavy scar tissue
- Women with very badly scarred or totally inaccessible cystic ovaries, making recovery of an egg impossible
- Women who do not ovulate in spite of treatment to stimulate the ovaries. For them, the only chance is to take an egg from another woman (see 'egg donation' later in this chapter)
- Women with such severe adhesions that collecting an egg would endanger their lives
- Women much over forty-two; experience has shown that beyond this age successful pregnancy seldom occurs after any fertility treatment
- Women whose ovaries respond very poorly when given drugs

to make them ovulate. These women, so-called 'poor-responders' are much more likely to be in the older age group.

THE STAGES OF TREATMENT

Careful assessment of your suitability for treatment is necessary first. This will include interviews with you and your partner. Because there are considerable stresses on you during treatment, responsible clinics try to make sure that you will be able to withstand the pressures that you may undergo. Most perform hormone tests to make certain the woman is capable of ovulating, the sperm count is checked carefully and a laparoscopy is usually needed before treatment to evaluate the ovaries. We feel that the uterine cavity should also be carefully assessed to make certain it is reasonably normal.

Stimulation of ovulation

At present, you have the best chance of success if more than one embryo is placed in your uterus. The chance of a pregnancy increases somewhat with more embryos but then, of course, there is also an increased risk of a multiple pregnancy with twins, triplets or even more babies.

In order to obtain more than one embryo, it is usual to give drugs to encourage the ovaries to produce more than one egg. Giving these drugs also has the advantage of improving the chance of collecting an egg at the best time. The drugs that are usually given are Clomid, or HMG (Pergonal or Humegon), but recently others have been tried, including FSH (see Chapter 3). In most units nowadays drug treatment with HMG or FSH is preceded by a course of drugs designed to damp down the pituitary gland, the so-called GnRH analogues (see Chapter 3). GnRH analogue treatment is often given in the form of a frequently sniffed nasal spray, or by injections. They are commonly given for 1–3 weeks before HMG injections are started. GnRH analogues result in a kind of temporary menopausal state which seems to encourage the ovaries to respond more actively when HMG injections are given. Consequently, more eggs are usually produced for the IVF process.

As soon as these drugs are stopped at the end of treatment, the 'menopausal' effect ceases and ovarian function returns to normal.

Egg collection

Ovulation normally occurs when the follicle grows to such a size that it bursts, usually when the follicle is about 1 in (2 cm) in diameter, on or about the fourteenth day of the cycle. At present, in vitro fertilization teams are really only able to work with mature eggs, and the egg is fully mature only about two to six hours before the follicle is due to burst. The egg is collected at this time by sucking out the follicle, just before it would be released. If the egg is obtained much earlier it cannot be fertilized, so a great deal of effort goes into the exact timing of this stage. Two kinds of tests can be used to time when ovulation will occur. Your doctors will use the method they have found the more reliable; most good units use both methods simultaneously, because the results of treatment are often improved. Moreover, the results of thorough regular hormone testing during a treatment cycle are useful to work out what went wrong after treatment has been unsuccessful.

Hormone tests   As the follicle increases in size before ovulation, the hormones estrogen and progesterone are produced in increasing quantities. Regular testing can detect this increase, preferably by blood tests, although a few clinics still test urine. In a normal untreated cycle, the pituitary gland in the brain also produces hormones, luteinizing hormone (LH) in particular, and this is a signal to the ovary to ovulate. Rising amounts of the hormone mean that ovulation will occur in the next twenty-four hours. Most IVF teams therefore give an injection of an LH-like hormone to stimulate ovulation at a precise and convenient time. This is usually in the form of HCG (human chorionic gonadotrophin; see page 46); if conditions are right, egg collection can be done between thirty-two and thirty-six hours later.

Ultrasound   The growth of the follicle can also be detected by ultrasound (see page 41). Ovulation is considered to be close when the largest follicle is bigger than 18 millimetres in diameter.

Once we are fairly certain that ovulation is about to happen, egg collection is planned. This can be done in two ways. Most clinics prefer to collect eggs using the ultrasound machine. After administration of a suitable local or general anaesthetic, the follicles are located by ultrasound, a needle is placed through the the wall of the vagina, and the eggs are sucked out. On rare occasions, when access to ovaries is difficult from below, the suction needle may be placed through the abdominal wall and thence into the ovary. An alternative method of egg collection uses the laparoscope, under general anaesthesia. The advantage of ultrasound is that it avoids this slightly bigger operation and in most centres only local anaesthetic is employed, allowing women to have egg collection on a day-care, outpatient basis. Whichever method is used and even with the greatest care in timing, we still very occasionally find that ovulation has already taken place. This usually means that it is impossible to collect eggs in that cycle and another attempt may be scheduled for a later month.

Egg culture, sperm preparation and fertilization

The eggs that have been collected are very easily damaged. They are identified under a microscope in the operating theatre and separated from the fluid surrounding them. They are then placed in specially prepared fluid, the culture medium, which contains precisely measured chemicals essential for continued survival of the egg. The eggs are then placed, in their culture medium, in an incubator, a sort of oven that keeps them at body temperature under similar conditions to the inside of your body.

While the eggs are being collected, your partner needs to have just produced a fresh semen sample. The sperm are washed in culture fluid and diluted. The number of sperm present is counted under a microscope. Approximately six hours after the egg has been collected, diluted sperm are placed in glass tubes, each containing one of the eggs. Within about forty-eight hours after mixing sperm and eggs together, the eggs are examined once or twice under a microscope to see whether they have been fertilized.

When a male fertility problem is suspected, various treatments to enhance the chance of fertilization may be used. For example, the sperm may be washed in a solution containing the drug Pentoxyfilline; this sometimes makes them more active. Alternatively, sperm injection may be used (see page 160).

Embryo culture

Usually by forty-eight hours, if the eggs have been fertilized, the embryo will have divided to form about four cells. Occasionally embryo growth may have advanced a little beyond this stage. If the embryos clearly look abnormal in any way, rather than chance the risk of a defective baby, they will be discarded.

Embryo transfer

At this stage, between two to four days after fertilization, embryos are ready to be put back into the uterus. They are loaded into a very fine piece of plastic tubing, together with the tiniest drop of culture fluid. You are put on a bed and the plastic tubing containing the embryos is very gently inserted through your cervix and into the uterus. A syringe is used to squirt the embryos into the uterus. This part of the procedure is painless, and nearly always done without an anaesthetic. Once the embryos have been transferred, you are usually asked to lie in bed for about thirty minutes. This appears to give the embryos a chance to stay put. A few units suggest that you stay in the hospital that night; most will allow you home immediately.

After transfer, nearly all women are nervous about what they can or cannot do. I do not feel that you should regard yourself as an invalid and there is no need to stay in bed, but it might be worth taking it easy for a few days. It may be best if you stay off work for two or three days and avoid having sex for two weeks. We have no evidence that even these simple precautions make much difference. I do strongly advise that overseas travel be avoided for two weeks, if possible.

Hormone treatment

Some teams think that the embryos have a better chance of implanting and forming a normal pregnancy if you are given progesterone after transfer, and for some days afterwards. You may be given injections of this hormone for a few days, or injections of HCG (see Chapter 3), which will stimulate your ovaries to produce more of it. This treatment is by no means universally used, though.

Pregnancy testing

Although embryo transfer may have gone very easily, the majority of embryos do not implant, but are shed or lost. Most clinics do a sophisticated blood test to see if there is any pregnancy hormone about one week after transfer, to discover whether a pregnancy is developing. The extremely disappointing result is that most women menstruate normally twelve to fourteen days after transfer, even though everything seemed to go just right.

WHAT ARE THE CHANCES OF A SUCCESSFUL PREGNANCY?

There are two particularly important factors affecting the chance of pregnancy after IVF. The first is the age of the woman. The second is whether or not there is more than one embryo available for transfer to the uterus.

Age Young women generally have a much better chance of success with IVF. In our own unit, women of thirty have a threefold greater chance than women of forty. Women who are over the age of forty are not only less likely to get pregnant after IVF, but if they do, are more likely to miscarry.

Number of embryos If you have had one embryo transferred, there is about an 8 to 18 per cent chance of a pregnancy depending on your age; if two embryos have been transferred, it's about 15 to 40 per cent. Although with three or more embryos transferred the chances may be better, there is a much greater chance of a multiple pregnancy, possibly triplets or more. Although having triplets may seem a special blessing if you are trying desperately to overcome your infertility, the risks are very serious. Miscarriage is much commoner, and premature delivery of very small, fragile babies is usual. A substantial number of triplets die, and most gynaecologists now agree that rigorous steps to prevent triplet pregnancy are needed. For this reason, nearly all IVF units limit the number of embryos they return to the uterus. Most in vitro fertilization programmes report that at least 10 per cent of their pregnancies are twins; this is, I feel, acccptable.

Success after repeated treatment

Of course, the treatment can always be repeated, but the chance of success is no higher the second time. Statistics at Hammersmith tend to show that if four good attempts have not resulted in a pregnancy, then your chance of success subsequently will actually be less. This may be because there is an undiagnosed problem preventing conception. Most clinics allow at least four attempts, though this varies from one to another; it depends also on your ability to stand the strain.

Why is the failure rate so high?

Unfortunately, even after women not suitable for IVF are excluded, it is full of pitfalls, and failure can occur at any one of these stages:

- The ovary may not respond properly to the stimulation. This occurs about 10 per cent of the time.
- Very occasionally, no eggs are obtained at egg collection. Sometimes ovulation has already happened by this time. This probably occurs in about 4 per cent of cases.
- Few or none of the eggs fertilize when mixed with the sperm. This happens in about 10 per cent of women treated.
- Some embryos fail to develop normally and are not suitable for embryo transfer. This happens about 20 per cent of the time.
- Embryo transfer is done but a pregnancy does not result. At present, only about 30 per cent or so of transfers in the best centres result in a pregnancy. We do not know yet why many apparently entirely satisfactory embryo transfers fail.
- The embryos implant but miscarry within a few weeks of treatment. This occurs in about 10 to 30 per cent of cases where pregnancy is achieved.

What are the risks of IVF?

The technique is not physically very risky. It is true that both ultrasonic and laparoscopic egg collection carry a small risk, but this is no greater than with other similar surgical procedures. In the normal course of events, laparoscopy may cause minor aches and pains in the chest and abdomen for about twenty-four to thirty-six hours after the anaesthetic. There is, rather surprisingly, another significant risk – that of ectopic pregnancy. After embryo transfer, the embryo may find its way into one of the tubes and implant there. This means an abdominal operation may have to be done to remove it (see Chapter 7). The risk of ectopic pregnancy varies from programme to programme, but it is not higher than about 6 per cent of pregnancies at worst. It is most common in women with tubal damage.

Overstimulation of the ovaries (see page 47) is an important complication, and is the result of the ovaries becoming very enlarged after HMG injections. This can cause pain and abdominal swelling, and occasionally necessitates admission to hospital before the ovaries return to their normal size. Overstimulation (or hyperstimulation syndrome, to give it its correct name) is seldom very serious, and usually settles within a few days or a week.

In truth, the worst risks of in vitro fertilization are really emotional and psychological.

Will you be able to stand the emotional strain?

There is no doubt that the main problem with in vitro fertilization is that it puts severe strain on the woman and, to a lesser extent, on her partner. This strain is often worse than the couple expects. The careful testing to time ovulation properly and the waiting time for egg collection and then embryo transfer requires fortitude. For the man, it may be difficult to masturbate and produce sperm when it is needed; the emotional tension at this moment is very considerable.

Once an embryo has been put back in the uterus, the situation is particularly fraught, because you are waiting so anxiously to see if a period will come on within the next two weeks. When embryos are transferred, it is only natural to feel 'emotionally pregnant', so when a period does come it is a cruel blow. This is bad enough, but should the period be delayed for a few days the shock can be catastrophic. This problem is a fact of treatment, and no couple should go in for in vitro fertilization unless they feel strong enough to withstand the anxiety involved. Having knowledge of these problems and understanding them beforehand is half the battle.

Will your baby be normal?

At the time of writing, only about 30,000 babies have been born as a result of IVF. About 6,000 of these births have been in the UK. There is no evidence of an increased risk of an abnormal baby from these pregnancies. The risk of any defect in normal pregnancies is about 1 in 80, and in vitro fertilization does not appear to increase it. Indeed, certain types of defect, such as an abnormality of the chromosomes, seem to happen less often than in the fertile population. There have been a few reports suggesting that IVF babies have, at birth, rather more birth problems than average. There are no hard data to support these reports and most gynaecologists feel that any worry on this score is simply because many people having IVF are in the older age group and need more general care during delivery. We have seen no serious problems at Hammersmith Hospital.

RECENT ADVANCES IN IVF

Freezing and storage of embryos

It is now possible to store embryos in a deeply frozen state, in liquid nitrogen. Providing freezing is carried out with proper care, human embryos appear to be capable of being stored at very low temperature for a considerable number of years. Following thawing, the embryo can be placed into the uterus, where it may give rise to pregnancy. This treatment may be helpful for women who, after having routine IVF treatment, have many spare embryos. Storing them for subsequent replacement means that another treatment will not involve the complexities of ovarian stimulation, monitoring and egg collection.

Embryo freezing has been widely promoted, and many patients believe that it is more successful than it really is. Current figures show that each single spare embryo frozen and stored has only a 2 to 3 per cent chance of producing a live baby after thawing and transfer. This is because not all embryos freeze successfully without damage, and frequently they do not survive thawing. Moreover, the fact that they appear normal after thawing by no means guarantees that they are viable. Thus several embryos may need to be transferred to get a reasonable chance of success, and that frozen/thawed embryo replacement may require repeated attempts.

Embryo freezing is quite a costly process and most clinics need to charge between £400 and £600 to cover the costs of long-term storage in liquid nitrogen. The evidence suggests that currently it is not as cost-effective as having fresh embryos transferred, because frozen embryo transfer may need repeated attempts (and therefore repeated costs) to have the same chance of pregnancy.

One concern about embryo freezing is that there are still questions in some doctors' minds about its complete safety. It is faintly possible that there are potential genetic risks to any children born after freezing. Although several hundred babies have now been born in Britain after embryo freezing, there has been no real follow up. Some doctors consider we cannot be sure, for example, that there is no risk to children, resulting from embryo freezing, of developing diseases such as leukaemia in later life. For the moment, therefore, my own feeling is that embryo freezing should only be used very cautiously.

In the near future, when the freezing technology is better understood and established, it will be possible not only to store embryos, but also eggs. At the present time egg freezing carries recognized risks of genetic damage. When we are able to freeze eggs safely, there will be great benefits for women who need egg donation.

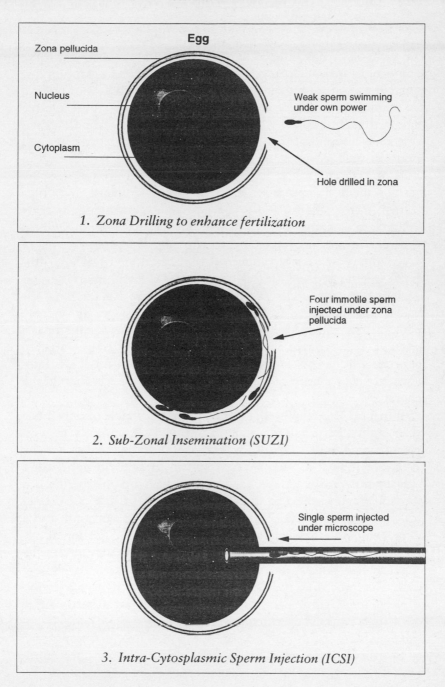

Egg

Zona pellucida

Nucleus

Cytoplasm

Weak sperm swimming under own power

Hole drilled in zona

1. Zona Drilling to enhance fertilization

Four immotile sperm injected under zona pellucida

2. Sub-Zonal Insemination (SUZI)

Single sperm injected under microscope

3. Intra-Cytosplasmic Sperm Injection (ICSI)

Sperm injection

IVF technology has resulted in a substantial break-through in the treatment of male infertility. IVF culture techniques have meant it is possible to culture human eggs in very small droplets of culture fluid containing concentrated numbers of sperm from an infertile male partner. Immediate access to eggs and sperm by laboratory scientisrs has also meant that it has been possible to prepare eggs and sperm in such a way as to increase the chance of fertilization in cases of male infertility. Sperms have been specially prepared by washing them in appropriate fluids or directly administering drugs to them in the culture, and prepared by such techniques as zona drilling (see diagram). But the biggest advance has been in the field of direct injection of sperm into the egg. Dr Simon Fishel of Nottingham University pioneered the technique of SUZI, Sub-Zonal Insemination. With this technique, Dr Fishel injects several sperm into the egg, under its outer protective covering, the zona pellucida. The technique requires a special microscope, fine micromanipulators and specially made microscopic glass needlesfor the injection. Because even slight unwanted movement can be a problem, the whole apparatus needs to be mounted on a specially designed heavy marble table which is isolated from vibration in the laboratory.

When SUZI is employed, even with sperm capable of only limited mortality, fertilization is much more likely. One problem with this approach is that because several sperm are injected under the zona, fertilization with several sperm in one egg (so-called 'polyspermy') is much more likely. Eggs which are polyspermic are not viable and have to be discarded; however, the use of SUZI in this way frequently results in just one sperm being successful and a normal embryo is formed. A recently developed modification of this technique involves injection of just one sperm directly under the zona and also directly into the substance (or cytoplasm) of the egg itself. This procedure is sometimes called DISCO (Direct Injection of Sperm into Cytoplasm of the Oocyte) or ICSI (IntraCystoplasmic Sperm Injection). The technique seems to have a significant advantage over SUZI in that polyspermic fertilisation does not occur.

In the past there have been questions as to whether direct injection into the egg may not run some risk of damaging it sufficiently seriously to cause an abnormality in any resulting foetus. Moreover, it is widely considered that many sperm which show poor motility may be genetically abnormal in some way. Clearly, it would be unwise to use any genetically damaged sperm to fertilise a human egg; the problem is that, at the present time, we have no way of detecting whether a poorly motile sperm is genetically defective or just simply sluggish.

Direct Sperm Injection (ICSI) has shown extreme promise over the last two years and there is now evidence that it is one of the most important treatments for male infertility. Several thousand babies have now been born in Europe, and many of the fears about the possibility of babies being born abnormal have now been dissipated. Many units, including our own, have consistently obtained a 25–30% success rate and direct sperm injection would therefore appear to be the most important advance in the treatment of male infertility in the last two decades.

EGG DONATION

Many women have premature menopause, often occuring in their twenties. This sad blow is serious, because it seems that their ovaries simply run out of eggs. As a result, menstruation stops, female hormone levels fall, and unless they have some form of hormone replacement therapy, they risk many of the problems associated with natural aging in much older women. Until recently, there was no possibility that such young women could become pregnant.

Great strides have been made in the last few years, using egg donation from altruistic donors. Eggs can be obtained from other women, fertilized with the patient's partner's sperm and then inserted into the women, just like normal IVF embryo transfer. The treatment requires that some form of hormone therapy be given first to the recipient, so that her uterus will be receptive. It has a very high degree of success; indeed, in our own unit almost 50 per cent of such procedures have been successful at the first attempt.

The problem is that egg donation is very difficult for the donor. Donors need to be carefully screened for genetic diseases and for conditions such as AIDS. They need to be relatively young women so that the risk of a chromosomally defective egg (causing such conditions as Down's syndrome) are minimized. The donor needs to undergo the kind of intensive ovarian stimulation that any IVF patient requires, with full monitoring – and all the inconvenience that involves. She needs an egg collection, requiring an operative procedure under some form of anaesthetic. Finally, and not least, she is giving her own unique genetic material. Under these circumstances it is understandable that egg donors do not readily come forward, and currently there is a severe shortage of this incredibly valuable material. In view of all these difficulties, it is not surprising that many units have widened their nets to try to obtain donors. For these reasons, some units are prepared to consider donation from relatives or friends of the donor. This is not without risk, however. The problem remains that 'known' donors may feel unusually possessive about any children which are conceived as a result of their considerable sacrifice. Until it is possible to store eggs by freezing, using similar technology as used for embryo freezing, donor eggs will remain a scarce resource. Once freezing of eggs is clearly established, it will be possible to get more of this material from women who are undergoing IVF for their own infertility problems.

GIFT TREATMENT AND UNEXPLAINED INFERTILITY

A discussion of in vitro fertilization would be incomplete without comment about GIFT treatment. GIFT was developed about twelve years ago and popularized by Dr Ricardo Asch and his colleagues in Texas. It has rapidly gained acceptance as a treatment, and there are now at least twenty or thirty centres in Britain which offer it. It involves simply taking an egg or eggs from the ovaries, sperm from the man, mixing them together and immediately placing them back into the woman. Replacement is not made into the uterus (unlike embryos during IVF) but into one or other fallopian tube. GIFT is an acronym, and stands for Gamete Intra-Fallopian Transfer – gametes being the eggs and sperm.

GIFT is different from IVF treatment, but has certain similarities. The main difference is that no attempt is made to produce an embryo outside the body, the eggs and sperm being simply mixed together in a drop of fluid and placed back into the body

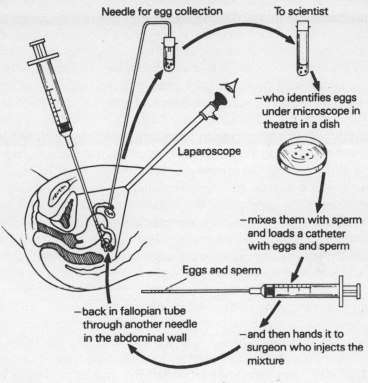

Needle for egg collection   To scientist

—who identifies eggs
under microscope in
theatre in a dish

Laparoscope

—mixes them with sperm
and loads a catheter
with eggs and sperm

Eggs and sperm

—back in fallopian tube
through another needle
in the abdominal wall

—and then hands it to
surgeon who injects the
mixture

The GIFT treatment

immediately. This avoids the need for the complex laboratory facilities required for IVF and for complicated artificial culture procedures (during which things can go wrong). Transfer of the egg/sperm mixture is done usually at the conclusion laparoscopy used to suck eggs from the follicles. The transfer is made by placing the mixture into one or other fallopian tube; this means the patient needs to have a normal tube remaining on one side for this to be possible. The main similarity is that laparoscopy has to be timed very carefully to take place just before ovulation, and that usually several eggs are collected simultaneously, to give a better chance of pregnancy. In order to get several eggs, drugs like clomiphene or HMG are given just as they are during IVF treatment. Most units using GIFT treatment are careful to limit the number of eggs they put back. The better and more successful doctors performing GIFT are usually prepared to put no more than four eggs into the tube. This is because there is a definite risk of multiple pregnancy (twins, triplets or more) if large numbers of eggs are replaced simultaneously.

GIFT is mainly considered useful for couples when absolutely no cause for the infertility can be detected, when there is mild endometriosis, or in some women when there is a persistent problem with the cervical mucus. GIFT has also been recommended by some doctors for treatment of male infertility, but it is not much more effective than simple timed insemination (Chapter 9), after stimulating the woman's ovaries with drugs to produce more than one egg. In fact, GIFT probably has very little or no value if the man is subfertile. GIFT should not be used if there is any evidence that your tubes have been damaged, or if you have previously had an ectopic pregnancy. This is because there is a real risk that inseminating the tube with the egg/sperm mixture could lead to another ectopic.

How successful is GIFT?

Some units claim that about one third of patients treated with GIFT have conceived. The truth is that, of course, some of these patients with unexplained infertility might have conceived naturally – without any treatment. GIFT also carries a slight risk of multiple pregnancy – for example, twins – because more than one egg is usually transferred simultaneously to the tube. One major problem with GIFT treatment is that if it doesn't work, you are really not much wiser. IVF has the advantage that it is to some extent diagnostic – the doctors can see whether your eggs have fertilized or not, and they can tell whether something is going wrong at the time of fertilization. The trouble with GIFT is that the eggs and sperm are put back before fertilization, and what happens to them after that cannot be observed and recorded. For this and other reasons, I am fairly convinced that GIFT will eventually be completely replaced by IVF, which is a much more informative and predictable treatment. Once we understand where the deficiencies are in the culture systems we are presently using for IVF and improve them, GIFT will be regarded as obsolete and will only be suitable for those patients who have religious or moral objections to the production of embryos by IVF therapy.

Other innovations include POST. POST, which stands for Peritoneal Ovum and Sperm Transfer, has been used in a few women. It involves the direct injection of sperm and eggs into the abdomen. To my mind it is unsafe, as it would appear to carry substantial risk of ectopic pregnancy. Fertility experts are fond of acronyms, and another recent one is DIPI – Direct Intraperitoneal Insemination. With this, sperm are injected through the wall of the vagina into the abdominal cavity. Claims are made that this treatment may be helpful when the man is not producing very fertile sperm, but the evidence for its value is a bit doubtful.

THE DIAGNOSIS OF 'UNEXPLAINED INFERTILITY'

An important word of caution. Far too frequently, patients are told that they are suffering from 'unexplained infertility' or 'idiopathic infertility'. To my mind the so-called diagnosis 'unexplained infertility' is clearly no diagnosis at all. It simply means that the doctors have failed to find out what is wrong. Unfortunately, it is a 'diagnosis' which is made far too frequently in most cases, frankly, because insufficient detailed tests have been done. A recent study of patients attending the Clinic at Hammersmith Hospital with a previous diagnosis of 'unexplained infertility' showed that over 80 per cent of them had not been completely investigated. Once proper tests had been completed in these couples, all that was often needed was fairly simple treatment, rather than GIFT or IVF.

The most common tests which tend to be omitted are:

- Adequate x-rays of the uterus which may show abnormalities not seen at laparoscopy in either your tubes or uterine cavity
- Hysteroscopy – telescope inspection of the inside of the uterus which may occasionally show abnormalities not seen otherwise (see page 87)
- Carefully timed post-coital testing to see if sperms are surviving in the cervix (page 96)
- Repeated sperm counts over several weeks or months to make certain there is no subtle abnormality (see page 131)
- Testing the sperm in special media – such as swim tests or

velocity testing – unfortunately these tests are not yet widely available (see page 133). However, when they are done, they often uncover a hidden cause for the supposed 'unexplained' problem
* Thorough hormone tests to detect abnormalities of male hormone or early falls in progesterone (see page 39)
* Scanning of the ovaries to see if follicles really are developing and there is no sign of polycystic ovaries (see page 41)

If you have been told that no cause can be found for your infertility, you should try to make sure that all the appropriate tests have been thoroughly done. Quite often, one or more of the tests above have not been completed. Before any involved treatment – GIFT, IVF or any other – try to make certain you are fairly satisfied that all possible tests that you can reasonably get done have been properly carried out. GIFT and IVF are particularly stressful major treatments and you should consider them only when they are really necessary.

THE ETHICAL PROBLEMS OF IN VITRO FERTILIZATION

Most people are concerned about the moral dangers of IVF. There are many issues involved, perhaps the most important of which is the status of the fertilized human egg. Do we doctors, having embryos produced by in vitro fertilization in our possession, have the right to discard them if they are surplus to our patients' needs? Should they be treated, as some would have it, like unborn children? Is it justified to perform research on human embryos?

Of course, there is a moral issue – few sensible people would deny that. Central to the issue is the status of the human embryo. People who are in favour of embryo handling and experiments argue that the embryos in question have not yet implanted in the uterus. They have no organs, no sensation and are a clump of undifferentiated cells. There is not even any guarantee that they would develop into babies. Indeed, hard evidence suggests that at least 40 per cent and possibly even 60 per cent of all human embryos do not implant, but are lost at the time of the next menstrual period. Certainly, nature herself does not offer the human embryo particular protection. The human embryo cannot even be said to have status as an individual at this stage (that is, up to fourteen days of development, when doctors agree that research should be stopped) as twins can form up to the fourteenth day of development.

People who wish to prevent work with human embryos point out that the beginning of human life can be regarded as the moment of fertilization. They argue that from that time the embryo has at least the potential to become a human being. They also argue that just because nature destroys embryos very readily, there is no reason for humans to do the same thing. They claim that evil scientists may wish to continue working with embryos long after the fourteen-day limit agreed by doctors; they suggest that a complete embargo on embryo research is the only way to prevent our society from starting to slide down a slippery slope.

Why embryo research is so important

What is undoubtedly true is that embryo research could prove to be of great human good. No IVF babies would have been born without it. All those thousands of healthy IVF babies now walking on the face of the globe would not have existed without the experiments that were needed to produce children like Louise Brown, the first IVF baby. The main reasons for embryo research are:

To improve existing infertility treatments for both male and female problems. It is depressingly true that only a proportion of infertile couples will have their own baby as a result of treatment. Otherwise there would be no need for books like this. Of course, embryo research is not the only form of research that is needed but it is undoubtedly one of the most important areas.

To investigate infertility when the cause is not clear. The need here is to take sperms from the man, eggs from the woman, mix them together and see why fertilization or embryo development doesn't happen. If there is no fertilization at all and no reason can be found, then at least the couple can be made fully aware of their situation. If allowed, such diagnostic techniques would be most helpful in reducing the great hardship and doubt infertile men and women experience.

To gain information about miscarriages About 100,000 women miscarry each year in the UK alone. Most of the time we have little or no idea why this happens (see Chapter 7). Many women miscarry repeatedly and suffer hugely in consequence. Research with embryos from couples like this is starting to provide great insight into what is going wrong. This kind of research will in time lead to an ability to transfer healthy embryos which are much less likely to miscarry.

To reduce genetic disease About 14,000 babies die each year as a result of genetic disease. A much larger number are born with handicaps that seriously affect their lives and the lives of their families. It would surely be better to prevent these genetic diseases, where possible. Embryo research has now resulted in the first healthy babies being born to families who had previously lost a child through genetic disease. A peculiar anomaly at present is that society regards it as perfectly acceptable to allow abortion at advanced stages of pregnancy if genetic disease is suspected. This is the termination of a pregnancy when the foetus is fully formed. It is surely preferable to reduce the need for abortion at all in such circumstances.

Opponents of embryo research contend that work with animal embryos is all that is required. Unfortunately, that is not true. Animal embryo research is indeed important, but human beings suffer from certain genetic diseases that are unique to them alone.

To improve contraception Although this area may seem of little interest to infertile couples, some of you reading this book may be infertile partly because of contraceptives that you have used. For example, the coil is known in certain cases to damage the uterine lining, and this may be permanent, resulting in subfertility. All methods of contraception have risks and side effects – none are perfect. There is a great need both to improve the existing methods and to develop safer, more effective drugs. Research on embryos is needed to make certain that none of the newer compounds would damage a baby conceived by someone who had been using them.

In summary, there seem to be overwhelming human arguments to continue research in these areas. Of course it is imperative that such work is properly controlled by governments, and at present this research is carefully licensed in the UK by the government body the Human Fertilization and Embryology Authority. Nobody wants to see Frankenstein experiments, even were these possible. However, many doctors agree that not to continue with such valuable work would be a disaster. It has been argued, I think correctly, that to discard embryos found to be 'spares' at the time of in vitro fertilization is far less ethical than doing properly supervised research with them.

11

Donor insemination, adoption and surrogacy

In this chapter I discuss possible alternatives for people who have found that their infertility is permanent and yet they still want desperately to have children. None of these options is easy, and to be successful both partners need commitment and fortitude. Each has similarities and requires somewhat similar decisions.

ARTIFICIAL INSEMINATION BY DONOR (AID)

Donor insemination is not a treatment for infertility. Rather it is an alternative. The decision to undergo AID is one that must be taken quite separately from routine infertility treatment. It is closer to adoption in many ways, and so needs similar considerations.

Artificial insemination may not appeal at first. There are many worries about it, and in this chapter I try to air some problems that people want to discuss about AID.

Is a child born as a result of AID at a disadvantage?

The biggest issue in AID treatment is whether an AID child may feel deprived or have other problems. To be truthful, there is insufficient information or detailed follow-up for us to be certain about the emotional problems that children born by AID may experience. What evidence there is suggests that AID children are concerned to know who their genetic father is, but that this does not cut across a loving relationship with the parents who have brought them up. One warning. It could be thought that, because there is doubt as to how a child may feel about being the result of AID, it is better that AID children should know nothing about their conception. I am sure that secrecy is wrong. Family secrets have a habit of coming out, often at moments of family quarrel or crisis. Revelations of this sort and against this background would be devastating for most children, and it must be preferable for them to understand how they were conceived as soon as they are able to comprehend the problem. The risks of not telling far outweigh the risks of honesty.

Is AID socially and emotionally acceptable?

The decision to go for AID is a very personal one, and nobody can tell you whether it is right for you and your relationship. At one level it is not so far removed from adoption, except that it has the enormous advantage that it is easier to obtain. Obviously it also means that you have the chance of rearing a child from the moment of conception, and that the child is genetically related to one of you. There is still a kind of stigma attached to AID which in some respects may be difficult to appreciate. Infertile couples may be quite happy about talking to their friends and parents about adoption; they may be much more reluctant to talk openly about plans for AID. This may cause all kinds of worries about prospective 'grandparents' and what they are told, for example. Certainly it is something the two of you will need to thrash out very carefully. Fortunately, the stigma (more imagined than real) around AID is disappearing. Although precise figures are difficult to obtain, it is reassuring to know that probably more than 10,000 AID babies have been born in Britain and more than 100,000 in the United States. AID is widely available in Australia and many other countries, especially in Europe, where it has been increasingly used for fifteen years. Very few problems with it have been reported. There is no evidence that children have suffered, providing the subject has been thoroughly discussed from the beginning and the child is aware of his or her background.

Sometimes couples think that a child born by AID will be less acceptable to the man than the woman. This also tends to be an imagined problem. There is no evidence that the male partner will not love and appreciate a child that is not genetically related to him – just as a genetic relationship with the father by no means guarantees a close relationship. One problem is that society has not yet fully come to terms with AID, although at least now most countries have taken steps to rectify some of the legal anomalies. At present, under English law, a child born as a result of AID is technically illegitimate and is supposed to be adopted by its social father. Birth certificates require the name of the biological father, but donors are usually anonymous, so many couples have to get round this by filling in false information. Strictly speaking this is perjury, although nobody has ever been prosecuted. Fortunately, it is now very likely that this legal anomaly will be changed because AID is so widely and increasingly accepted.

Will my partner love an AID child?

This is a question the woman sometimes asks me. In my experience, this is rarely a problem. The male partner becomes closely involved and shares the pregnancy and birth. If the decision to have AID is taken mutually and freely discussed, his relationship with the child need be no different from those of other children with their fathers. As it seems that the growing environment has a lot more influence than blood relationship, your child will rapidly take on the characteristics and outlook of your partner and so he will be as deeply involved in parenthood.

How is AID done?

Donor insemination is done in a similar way to insemination with your partner's semen (see Chapter 9). It is important that it is done just before ovulation. This may require ultrasound tests and even blood tests to make certain that you are inseminated at the best time. Some clinics also give a small dose of clomiphene, the drug that encourages you to ovulate at a definite time.

Should the woman's fertility be tested first?

Opinions vary about how much investigation the woman should have before attempting donor insemination. I feel that if there is no obvious reason from a woman's history for infertility, it is reasonable to try AID, but limiting it to three cycles. If no pregnancy has occurred by then, careful tests are needed, perhaps including laparoscopy.

When there is nothing wrong with the woman or the sperm, AID will result in a pregnancy in 35 per cent of women after about four cycles. Around 90 per cent will conceive after about one year, providing the sperm is really satisfactory, you are fertile and the technique is being carried out properly. If you get pregnant, the pregnancy should be entirely normal and the risk of miscarriage is no greater than it is for any normal pregnancy.

Obtaining donor insemination

Donors, who usually remain anonymous, are chosen because they have a good sperm count. Most clinics use volunteer medical students. Of course, because they are often not yet married it is not known if they are fertile even though they have an adequate sperm count. Occasionally donor insemination fails because there is something wrong with the sperm that does not show on testing. If several inseminations fail, the doctor will switch to a different donor.

Donors are usually matched for the more simple characteristics of your partner, such as general build, colouring and ethnic background. This tends to ensure that any child resembles your partner. Most clinics confirm too that their blood groups are compatible. Donors are also screened for genetic disease and infections that may harm the woman. We feel that donors must be carefully screened for dangerous viruses, such as the AIDS virus, as well. This carries certain difficulties at present because of the theoretical risk that the donor may be incubating the virus, but testing may be negative at this very early stage. Semen may be inseminated fresh, within about two hours of masturbation. Alternatively, frozen semen may be used. This is much more convenient, as it can be collected at any time, processed and placed in liquid nitrogen where it will retain its fertility for many years. All that is needed is for the semen to be thawed, which takes about twenty minutes. There is no evidence that semen freezing carries any risk of abnormality for the foetus, so there is no need to be worried on this front.

How can you get AID?

Because male infertility is so unpredictable and many men with poor counts end up producing a pregnancy, the majority of doctors are quite reluctant to offer AID. This means that you may have to bring the subject up with your doctor first. He or she may want you to try AID only as a last resort.

In most parts of the world it is available only on a private basis. Repeated cycles of treatment tend to be expensive, so it may be wise to make as certain as possible that there is no major problem with the woman first. In England, there are a few clinics that offer a free service. These mostly take on women who have been carefully screened and who are in a regular relationship. AID will be offered only after lengthy discussion with both partners and after signed consent. If you are finding it difficult to discover where AID is available, contact one of the infertility support groups listed at the end of this book.

AID and AIDS

One recent worry, which has concerned many people, is the risk of catching the Human Immunodeficiency Virus (HIV or AIDS) from donor semen. Recently, the American Fertility Society in the USA and the Royal College of Obstetricians and Gynaecologists in Britain have laid down guidelines to avoid this risk. The American guidelines which should be used by all physicians undertaking donor insemination in North America were published in the Society's official journal *Fertility and Sterility* in October, 1986 (Volume 46, 4, pages 95S–109S). Similar guidelines are used in Britain. They include the careful monitoring and repeated testing of all donors. Many doctors also prefer to use only frozen semen which is stored for a minimum of three months after the donor's serologic tests for AIDS are negative. You should confirm with your doctor that any semen being employed has been collected according to the criteria laid down by the Royal College of Obstetricians and Gynaecologists or, in the USA, by the American Fertility Society.

ADOPTION

Perhaps the most important thing to remember before going for adoption is that it is necessary to come to terms with your infertility. There will have to be a period of grief and mourning before you see adoption as a positive alternative.

Unfortunately, adoption is extremely difficult nowadays. Estimates of the numbers of infertile couples vary, but there are likely to be well over 600,000 in the United Kingdom alone. Against that figure only about 950 babies under six months are adopted each year. Several thousand more, older children, are adopted by infertile couples annually, but it is probable that only one in ten infertile couples who apply receive a baby each year. It can also be surprisingly difficult to obtain advice. Few doctors dealing with infertility have much feeling about adoption and many more tend to shrug off a couple's problem – the attitude is 'Well, you can always adopt.' In fact, because of the huge difficulties involved, adoption is a viable alternative only for a tiny minority of couples.

Are you eligible for adoption?

Adoption agencies vary widely in their criteria. Most will not consider single parents at all. Normally, an adoption agency expects couples to have been married for at least three or four years; they may be less likely to consider an application from you if you have been previously divorced. They are also less likely to consider applications from people who have been married for a very long time as it is felt that a childless couple who have been together for longer than ten or twelve years may be unable to adjust easily to the demands of a young child. Age is another factor. Very few agencies will consider couples where either partner, but especially the woman, is much over thirty-five. Nor may they consider your application if there is a big age difference between you and your partner. It is wise at an early stage to consult your local authority social service department.

Most agencies will consider your application only if you have given up fertility treatment entirely. The main reason is to ensure that the couple have come to terms with their infertility. Some agencies therefore ask for written confirmation from the family doctor or gynaecologist that the couple are irrevocably infertile and that no further treatment is possible. Most specialists are very happy to give such letters to infertile couples – even if they have a sneaking suspicion that there may be more treatment around the corner. This is partly because no doctor can predict what new treatments may be developed and partly because no matter how infertile you are, miracles do occasionally happen and it is not unknown for an adopting woman to conceive within a few months of adoption. On this subject, however, there is no substance in the myth that if you adopt you are more likely to conceive spontaneously.

Adoption agencies expect both partners to be in reasonably good physical shape. They usually want certification from your family doctor that you have no serious disease – you will probably have to undergo a medical examination. They may also ask for a letter from your specialist confirming that the condition causing your infertility is of no risk to your general health. For example, this may be the case if you have blocked tubes as a result of old tuberculosis. Adoption agencies are responsible for ensuring that the children available for adoption are healthy as well and they will have a full medical history for the child and his or her parents. A thorough general examination of the baby will have been carried out and specialist paediatric advice sought. For this reason it is not wise to use an unknown or untried source offering a child for adoption. Some people, in their anxiety to adopt, are tempted to go out of their country for an infant. There is no information about the child's origins or health in many of these cases and the risks of later trouble are not generally worth taking. Furthermore, private arrangements, adoption by means of a third party placing, are no longer legal in the UK.

Adoption agencies will take your social background into account. Obviously they are mostly concerned to make sure your partnership is stable. Most will look at your income and your home, and you will need to demonstrate that you can care materially for a child.

By now you will realize that adoption demands considerable commitment. Adoption agencies vary hugely. You may find their attentions and those of social workers intrusive and unpleasant – especially after you have just gone through the emotional hassle of lengthy and unsuccessful infertility treatment. Many couples, for example, find it extremely distressing to answer the intimate questions asked by some social workers about their sex lives. Alternatively, you may find the people with whom you come in contact extremely sympathetic and helpful. While some offer little in the way of counselling, others give you very thorough counselling and advice. Agencies also vary in policy. For instance, some may be perfectly happy for you to continue with infertility tests, while others may regard this as an absolute bar to adoption.

What are the emotional problems?

First, adoption will require as much from your partner as from you. You will both need to be heavily involved, even if *he* was relatively unenthusiastic or distanced himself during the infertility tests. This you will need to work out if, for example, your partner does not feel the grief of infertility as badly as you do. You must both appear committed and positive in front of everyone involved with the adoption. This need to prove your commitment may cause resentment if you are both convinced that you would be admirable parents and have seen others whom you consider less than ideal. You will simply have to swallow any resentment and be prepared to be quite open about what have been very private feelings.

Going for adoption means that you are opting to rear a child rather than bear one. For some people the actual state of being pregnant is crucially important. Some women feel deeply that a part of life has escaped them because they have not gone through pregnancy and childbirth. For them, adoption may not be a good solution. Although the act of giving birth has been shown to be important in bonding, women who adopt successfully do not find that their relationship with their child is any less loving than that of other mothers. Nevertheless, some adopting mothers continue to feel a longing for actually having given birth to their adopted children.

Neither you nor your partner are genetically related to your adopted child. For many people, having a child is the ultimate fusion of their relationship together. Their being and personalities are united in their child. They may be worried about adopting as the child is not directly the result of their life together. Others worry about the different physical characteristics, but there is a curious irony here. Remarkably frequently you will find that acquaintances compliment you on the appearance of your adopted child, commenting on how he or she takes after one of you.

One set of emotions you may not be prepared for or warned about are those that you may have on the arrival of your adopted child. This can reawaken feelings of grief over infertility, emotions to which you thought you had become adjusted. This grief is an expression of your inability to bear 'your own' child and can be quite startling. You may feel guilty about this, particularly at a time when you are trying to establish a relationship with your adopted child. As that relationship develops the grief will gradually disappear.

What about the child?

Research has shown that, contrary to many people's fears, adopted children turn out to be well-adjusted and stable as well as normally intelligent. Obviously, all parents – fertile ones included – worry about how their children will develop. There is not the slightest evidence that adopted children are worse off.

Your child has the right and the need to know that he or she is adopted. Legally nowadays, at late adolescence, the child has the right to find out who the genetic parents are. You must be ready to deal with your child's discovery of two sets of parents. This should not create any longterm difficulty. Research has shown that children who know who their genetic mother is generally have little desire to make contact with her. If they do, it is to get more than just a mental picture of her. They want to know how she is now and how life has treated her. This curiosity is natural, and does not reflect on the adopting parents and their loving relationship with their child.

How do you go about adoption?

First find a sound source to discuss and consider this action. Some local authorities can be most helpful. Write to as many of your local adoption agencies as you can. If you are religious, you should mention that, but do not apply to religious adoption agencies if you are not a regular churchgoer. There are more children from ethnic minorities available for adoption. If you are prepared to adopt an older child, or a child with certain problems, you may find adoption easier – so that is worth remembering when you write your letter. Bear in mind too that letters are not always answered and it is worth writing repeatedly if you do not get an answer immediately.

If you get to the next stage, you will probably be asked to attend meetings to find out more. You may meet people who have already adopted and others, like yourselves, who are going through the process. Discussion may help you decide whether this course of action is really for you. After this comes the long process of talking with social workers and eventually the chance to have your baby or child when available.

SURROGACY

Surrogacy has recently become topical. It has been suggested for couples where the female partner is absolutely infertile – for example, she has no uterus. Basically, it means a fertile woman having a baby for another. The baby is handed over to the infertile woman at birth. There are two sorts of surrogacy:

1. The woman who is to give birth, the surrogate, is inseminated with sperm from the husband of the infertile wife. There are well-documented cases where the husband has actually had intercourse with the fertile woman, the arrangement being that the baby is handed over at birth.

2. The second type always requires help from a doctor. It involves taking an egg from the infertile woman (assuming, of course, that she is capable of producing eggs) and taking sperm from

her husband. An embryo is produced using IVF, and this embryo is placed in the uterus of a surrogate mother who has agreed to hand the baby over to the infertile woman after birth.

A theoretical advantage of the second type of surrogacy is that the child is genetically the child of the infertile couple, as the egg came from the 'adopting' mother. In effect, the surrogate mother – the woman who gave birth – is unrelated to the child. A clear disadvantage is that it requires all the technology of test-tube baby treatment and considerable medical intervention.

What are the problems of surrogacy?

My feeling is that surrogacy of any sort is fraught with dangers. Recognition of this is clear in recent legislation in the UK, which has made any form of surrogacy involving a commercial transaction illegal. This means that surrogacy agencies are against the law in Britain. Surrogacy is also illegal in Australia, but not yet in the United States. Irrespective of legal issues, it seems to me that there are a number of human arguments that question the wisdom of surrogacy. They include:

The risks to the surrogate mother, who is expected to give up her child after the increasing attachment formed during pregnancy. Even if a woman starts her pregnancy full of the altruistic desire to give the baby to another woman who desperately wants one, she will most likely find giving up the baby extremely damaging emotionally when the time comes.

The risks to the child   There is always the problem of secrecy. If the surrogate arrangement is kept secret from the child, there is the profound risk that he or she may find out about his origins inadvertently, perhaps at the height of a family quarrel or other crisis. Such an appalling shock might well be permanently damaging. If the surrogate arrangement is not kept secret, the child could harbour strong feelings of love towards his or her surrogate mother, and possibly negative feelings towards the adopting mother. This could produce severe emotional problems for both mothers.

The risks for the adopting parents   The child's mother may always feel guilty and inferior because her child has not been given birth by her. The father may harbour unexpressed or ill-suppressed affection for the bearing mother at the expense of his partner.

The legal difficulties   Many areas remain unresolved legally. Who takes responsibility if the surrogate mother is ill as a result of the pregnancy? Who looks after the child if it is born with a defect? What rights does the surrogate mother have if she refuses to hand the baby over to its adopting parents (bearing in mind the father is the biological father)?

Clearly, surrogacy is a minefield, and immense difficulties face people who consider it as an answer to their infertility. While I am strongly opposed to making surrogacy itself illegal, I feel that the British Parliament was right to make surrogacy involving financial arrangements a criminal offence because of the risks of exploitation of both the woman concerned and the child. Despite my grave reservations regarding every aspect of surrogacy, I admit that I feel that there are certain very rare situations where it may be a perfectly reasonable option.

12

Dealing with untreatable infertility – Sources of further help

There comes a point in your life when infertility can become extremely corrosive. So often, I find myself sitting in front of couples who feel that all their values have become corrupted. Unless you take very careful stock, your anguish and bitterness can destroy all the good potential of your life. How do you cope?

In many ways it seems presumptuous for someone like myself, without the personal experience of childlessness, to offer advice. I have felt deeply, though, about the many thousands of couples who have enriched my thinking about childlessness; in some ways I find it an advantage to be slightly outside the problem. Different couples cope with childlessness in different ways, but here are some general points that may help if you have recently been told that there is no further treatment possible.

- Learning of failed treatment or failed adoption procedures comes as a bitter blow and a real shock for everyone, no matter how well prepared in advance. This may be the time to consider the cut-off point, a recognition of your situation. Resolution of your sadness at being infertile may come only if you grieve, if you really cry. A period of mourning can be the most constructive way to get over untreatable infertility. Once the uncertainty of your situation is resolved, you can begin to live again.

- Stop thinking of the possibility that you may miss your next period. When you are infertile, each menstrual period can be a shock, particularly if you are expecting to miss it. You may be one of the unfortunate people who have irregular, painful or delayed periods, and this makes things much more difficult. Some infertile women find it helpful deliberately to avoid recording the dates of their periods or keeping any form of menstrual diary.

- Stop worrying about the past. It doesn't help to think about an infection that you fear you may have neglected, or to dwell on an abortion that was necessary at a time when your whole situation was quite different. Nor does it help to keep remembering the operation that you turned down until it was too late to do anything about it. Your reasons were better than they may appear to you now, and it is utterly destructive to think how you might have handled things differently.

- Try to find a cause for your infertility – and then forget it. If you cannot find the cause, you have to accept that in some cases no cause can be found. Continued speculation can lead to feelings of guilt or blame. This can make your relationship with your partner less satisfactory at a time when it needs to be at its strongest.

- Stop feeling guilty. Just remember that every infertile person, man or woman, feels guilty at some stage. The guilt seldom, if ever, has any bearing on reality. In my experience, infertility is never anyone's fault – just as catching influenza or developing cancer is no one's fault. You may be in some way reassured to know that many cancer sufferers also experience deep feelings of guilt – which, of course, are equally illogical.

- Try to accept that you have done everything possible. This may be more difficult if the doctors you have been seeing are continuing with half-hearted treatments. It is worth asking yourself – and them – whether you have now reached the stage where you have done everything. This requires courage, because you may not really want to hear the answer. However, unless you face this you will find it very difficult to resolve your problems.

- Try not to let your feelings bubble over too much with friends. While it is good to get to the point where you feel far more open about your infertility, continued reference to your problems may prove an unwelcome burden to some friends, though not to others. Judge where you stand, because your friendships are specially important to you now.
- Ignore the press and especially its banners of new developments in infertility. Headlines such as 'Revolutionary treatment brings new hope for infertile couples' very seldom in my experience have any real foundation. Infertility, especially when it concerns human embryos, sells newspapers and television programmes. Don't allow yourself to be indirectly exploited by the media. Remain healthily sceptical about success rates claimed in the press – they are invariably over-optimistic.
- Ask yourself whether you have a chance to develop another aspect of your life. If you are not bringing up children you are likely to have more time on your hands than many of your friends. If you have a job, it may be worth thinking whether there is more you can put into it. Hobbies, your home, friendships or voluntary service are other areas where many infertile women find ways of making a radical change in their lives.
- Communicate with your partner. Your best support is likely to be your partner. Work out how you can spend more time doing things together. Your sex life is most likely to have taken quite a battering and you should re-evaluate how sex could become a pleasure once again, rather than an unspontaneous chore.

SUPPORT GROUPS

It is comparatively recently that there has been much awareness of the needs of the infertile. Many of the larger infertility clinics have encouraged the formation of support groups, which tend to help infertile couples get in touch with each other and to hold group meetings. Some of these groups help raise money for the more esoteric treatments, such as in vitro fertilization. I think that they perform a useful function and the interaction between couples can be comforting. You may consider starting such a group in your local clinic. It may be worth asking the consultant in charge for his or her approval and advice. One group I know of has regular monthly meetings, produces a newsletter and raises sums of money which go to improve such amenities as outpatient facilities.

On a more official basis are the national organizations. In the UK the first, CHILD, was founded in the late 1970s. It is devoted purely to improving facilities for infertile people, developing counselling and promoting research. CHILD produces a newsletter called *Childchat* which contains information about new treatments, a doctor's advice column, letters from patients and regular features from leading medical specialists. CHILD also has a hotline for distressed people, and you are encouraged to telephone this number if you want a chat. CHILD holds regular group meetings, usually in private houses, to which speakers on different subjects concerned with infertility are invited.

The second British organization is ISSUE (formerly called NAC, the National Association for the Childless, founded in 1976). This is a larger organization than CHILD and does not cater only for infertile people, as some of its members are voluntarily childless. It, too, does excellent work with a heavy accent on counselling. Indeed, NAC's founder, Peter Houghton, has co-written a recommended book on the emotional aspects of infertility (see page 190). ISSUE brings out a series of leaflets, which are regularly updated, on differing infertility treatments. Like CHILD, ISSUE produces a newsletter. In recent years NAC has organized highly successful national meetings on the wider implications of infertility. Expert speakers and good organization have been the hallmark of these annual events.

I would offer one word of caution. Both CHILD and ISSUE seem to me to be somewhat obsessed with in vitro fertilization. I feel that both organizations lay too much emphasis on this treatment, while other much more important and more successful infertility treatments are neglected. (Both addresses are on page 191.)

A third British organization, which is not really a support group at all, is PROGRESS. This is concerned with the protection and promotion of research into all aspects of human reproduction. The main thrust of that research is infertility, and the organization really cares that infertile people get a better deal. It has strong

Parliamentary connections and is there to make sure that any legislation on such matters as embryo research, infertility treatments and IVF is not to the detriment of childless couples. If you have an interest in the legal aspects of infertility or an interest in promoting better research, you should join.

13

Ten points for infertile couples

1. Infertility is not a disease. It is a symptom. It is a medical principle that before a symptom is treated, the cause must be found first. Therefore, make certain that you are not being given treatment before reasonable attempts have been made to find the cause of your infertility.

2. Make certain that you understand both the purpose of each test you have and the results. Try to get a fairly clear idea of the reason for any proposed treatment so that you know what is expected of you, how to proceed and – most important – you feel that you have participated in your treatment.

3. Although it is reasonable to seek a second opinion, or to ask to be seen at a specialist centre for a treatment that is not available locally, be careful not to 'hawk around'. Endless changes and visiting different doctors will only ensure that you get different opinions and conflicting treatment. Hawking around is in effect denying resolution of your problems.

4. For tests to be significant, they must be conducted under proper conditions. Do not get depressed about a single negative post-coital test, a low sperm analysis, a single low hormone

result or a failed cycle with clomiphene. One swallow doesn't make a summer – one snowflake doesn't mean it's winter.

5. If you are offered treatment that is not of proven value, such as pills to improve sperm count, pills to improve post-coital tests or methods of timing intercourse, think carefully. By all means try them, but remember that they are speculative and their use may damage your sense of well-being. Set a time limit on them and resolve to stop them when that time is up.

6. One treatment that can be particularly upsetting to infertile couples is artificial insemination with the husband's sperm. If this is being considered, ask yourself what you expect to achieve. It tends to be offered when the doctor has nothing more concrete to give. It is sexually invasive and often demoralizing. Remember that except in very specific circumstances, you and your husband are just as capable of getting enough sperm to the right place without any interference. You are certainly likely to enjoy this more.

7. Remember that very few infertility treatments produce immediate results. It takes, on average, five months for a normally fertile couple to achieve pregnancy. If you are infertile, your various systems will not be working so efficiently and it will probably take you longer. This is especially true after tubal surgery or if the sperm count is abnormal. With low sperm counts, the best chance may just be to allow time, by continued exposure to the chance of pregnancy. Although this is difficult to adjust to, there is nearly always some hope.

8. Please remember that IVF really is the last resort. The ludicrous publicity surrounding it has undoubtedly distracted attention from much more important treatments, which are cheaper, more successful and less emotionally demanding. There is a serious risk that the attention given to IVF will delay improvements in other infertility services which are far more important.

9. AID and adoption are frequently seen as a kind of treatment

for infertility. They are not. They both require a reappraisal of your situation, your attitudes and your aspirations. Even though AID is carried out in a medical environment, it raises many of the issues of adoption and the medical aspects are incidental.

10. Infertility has many negative and destructive aspects. It can also have the positive effect of strengthening and improving your partnership or your marriage. Do your best to ensure that it enhances the positive aspects of your life.

Books on infertility

The following is not a comprehensive list. I have chosen mainly from the most recent publications, and I have limited myself to a few books which I feel are most useful and have broken new ground.

The Experience of Infertility, Naomi Pfeffer and Anne Woolett (Virago Press, London, 1983)
This is an admirable book, written from a strongly feminist viewpoint. It is exceptionally good on the feelings that infertile couples have – better on female than male feelings. It is also valuable for its realistic attitude towards IVF. Its main weakness is that it is not particularly accurate medically, and the evaluation of the various tests described is often accompanied by misleading information. Nevertheless, the sensitivity of the authors makes this a book that I feel should be read.

Coping with Childlessness, Diane and Peter Houghton (Unwin Paperbacks, London, 1987)
Another good book, which focuses on the emotions roused by infertility. It is written with a sense of humour, and I think it would be emotionally healing for any infertile couple who read it. It is also admirably critical of the advice and counselling that infertile people get. Its weakness is the description of the medical and investigative aspects of infertility, which is reasonably accurate but

quite inadequate. However, for my money this is one of the most valuable and sensitive publications on severe infertility that I have read.

Coping with a Miscarriage, Hank Pizer and Christine O'Brien Palinski (Jill Norman, London, 1980)
This deals with the medical and emotional aspects of miscarriage and is written by a doctor and someone with personal experience of repeated miscarriages. It contains a good deal of information, not all up-to-date, and some useful references.

The Gift of a Child, R. Snowden (George Allen and Unwin, London, 1984)
This is a digestible and easily read account of the problems concerned with AID. It is a useful examination of the issues involved and will be helpful to many thinking of this solution.

Everything you need to know about Adoption, Maggie Jones (Sheldon Press, London, 1987)
A guide to adoption which is simply and clearly expressed.

Adopting a Child: A Brief Guide for Prospective Adopters (British Agencies for Adoption and Fostering, 1984)
This is really a pamphlet which has been updated annually. It is a most useful although brief introduction and is essential reading if you are considering this course of action. It contains a useful list of the agencies to contact in England and Wales.

USEFUL ADDRESSES

CHILD
01424 73236

ISSUE
509 Aldridge Road, Great Barr, Birmingham B44 8NA
0121 344 4414

Index